In North America there is much public interest in and cost associated with health and medicine. *The Biblical Guide to Alternative Medicine* addresses the subject from a balanced biblical worldview. This includes recognizing God and Jesus as the source of wholeness, while acknowledging spiritual forces of darkness that oppose health. Individuals need to assume responsibility for their physical, psychological and especially their spiritual health. Faulty and potentially dangerous medical systems are analyzed and exposed. I recommend this book to health-care professionals, pastors and laymen.

GEORGE A. HURST, M.D., FACP, FCCP

DIRECTOR EMERITUS AND FORMER CHIEF ADMINISTRATIVE OFFICER
UNIVERSITY OF TEXAS HEALTH CENTER AT TYLER
CHAIRMAN OF THE BOARD FOR MINISTRY OF HEALING

I love the five-point grid set forth in this book that can help anyone assess various health practices. In the First Place program we seek to give God first place in every area of our life. We also believe that a balanced life brings life and health in all four areas—spiritual, mental, emotional and physical. The authors have done a great deal of research and present a compelling case for seeking God's will before undergoing any medical treatment. They also have researched the history of medicine and the pharmaceutical industry and give practical advice to those who are seeking God's best for their own personal health.

CAROLE LEWIS

FIRST PLACE NATIONAL DIRECTOR
HOUSTON, TEXAS

Health out of balance is a plague that is sweeping the Christian community. Because we have made health a god, we seek costly remedies that not only do not help but also can be spiritually destructive. Every Christian family needs this book to evaluate their health choices.

DR. JIM LOGAN

DIRECTOR OF I.C.B.C. OF IOWA
DEAN OF INTERNATIONAL MINISTERIAL INSTITUTE

I found this book by Neil T. Anderson and Michael Jacobson most informative and helpful. They have accumulated an enormous amount of history, science and biblical guidelines to direct one toward plausible avenues for health and recovery. What an advantage this information gives in avoiding so many futile healing adventures!

REX RUSSELL, M.D.

AUTHOR, *WHAT THE BIBLE SAYS ABOUT HEALTHY LIVING*
BSAHEALTHYLIVING.COM

The Biblical Guide to

ALTERNATIVE MEDICINE

NEIL T. ANDERSON

MICHAEL D. JACOBSON

Regal

From Gospel Light
Ventura, California, U.S.A.

PUBLISHED BY REGAL BOOKS
VENTURA, CALIFORNIA, U.S.A.
PRINTED IN THE U.S.A.

Regal

Regal Books is a ministry of Gospel Light, an evangelical Christian publisher dedicated to serving the local church. We believe God's vision for Gospel Light is to provide church leaders with biblical, user-friendly materials that will help them evangelize, disciple and minister to children, youth and families.

It is our prayer that this Regal book will help you discover biblical truth for your own life and help you meet the needs of others. May God richly bless you.

For a free catalog of resources from Regal Books/Gospel Light, please call your Christian supplier or contact us at 1-800-4-GOSPEL *or* www.regalbooks.com.

Cover and interior design by Robert Williams
Edited by Amy Simpson

Library of Congress Cataloging-in-Publication Data
Anderson, Neil T., 1942-
   The Biblical guide to alternative medicine / Neil T. Anderson   Michael
Jacobson.
        p. ; cm.
Includes bibliographical references and index.
   ISBN 0-8307-3083-4
   1. Alternative medicine. 2. Alternative medicine—Religious
aspects—Christianity. 3. Holistic medicine—Religious
aspects—Christianity.
   [DNLM: 1. Complementary Therapies—Popular Works. 2. Bible—Popular
Works. 3. Religion and Medicine—Popular Works.   WB 890 A5483b 2003]
I. Jacobson, Michael. II. Title.
   R733 .A555 2003
   615.5—dc21   2002014214

1 2 3 4 5 6 7 8 9 10 11 12 13 14 15 / 09 08 07 06 05 04 03 02

Rights for publishing this book in other languages are contracted by Gospel Light Worldwide, the international nonprofit ministry of Gospel Light. Gospel Light Worldwide also provides publishing and technical assistance to international publishers dedicated to producing Sunday School and Vacation Bible School curricula and books in the languages of the world. For additional information, visit www.gospellightworldwide.org; write to Gospel Light Worldwide, P.O. Box 3875, Ventura, CA 93006; or send an e-mail to info@gospellightworldwide.org.

CONTENTS

Part 1—*A Biblical Grid for Evaluating Medical Treatments*

Part 2—*Evaluating Medical Systems*

Part 3—*Evaluating Alternative Therapies*

Part 4—*To Your Good Health*

FOREWORD

Finally! Here is the book I have been searching for years to find. One that fully examines the many different approaches to health and explains the various forms of alternative medical practices from a solid Christian perspective. The book takes into consideration the whole person—body, soul and spirit—because our mind and emotions have so much to do with the degree of wholeness and health we enjoy. Along with many results of scientific testing, the historical roots of each practice are explained, as well as the religious system each practice is based on. Any unholy alignment by its founder, or those who practice it, is exposed as it is held up to the light of biblical truth.

With more choices now than ever before in the area of health and wellness, we must be able to discern which ones are from God and which are not. I know what it's like to be so sick and miserable that I was desperate to try anything that might bring relief. When people experience this degree of misery, they will reach out for whatever promises to alleviate their suffering. In the process, however, they can waste time and money on things that not only do not work but also may actually be harmful.

We don't want to be involved in a wrong health practice. And we don't want to wait until we are desperate before we try new medical practices about which we are not educated. We want the truth now so that we won't place our hope in a treatment that is not consistent with God's Word. We want to know the options available to us so that we can make wise choices, instead of expensive mistakes. This book will clear up much confusion on this subject and will be one of those balanced and solid books that you keep referring to whenever you have a question about your health. The information on these pages required a tremendous amount of research, and I'm grateful that Neil Anderson and Michael Jacobson did it all for me, so now I don't have to. I know you'll feel the same way as you sit back and benefit from their hard work.

Stormie Omartian
Author, *Greater Health God's Way* and *The Power of a Praying* series

INTRODUCTION

When I (Neil) was pastoring a church, I recall how excited I was to hear that a neighboring medical school was going to start a new program that would graduate family practitioners. The goal was to become more wholistic, with the new curriculum addressing nutritional as well as spiritual and psychological needs. My enthusiasm was quickly dampened, however, when I discovered that the spirituality being taught did not represent orthodox Christianity. Without divine revelation, the spiritual input took on the early forms of what we now understand to be New Age. Big names in medicine like Elizabeth Kubler-Ross and Jonas Salk soon found themselves taken in by the occult.

Christians should have been the ones promoting wholistic medicine, but instead it was the spirituality of New Age practitioners that stole the day. By the mid-1980s, many would have considered you a New Ager if you espoused wholistic health. Since that time, the interest in spirituality as a component of medicine has grown considerably. According to the George Washington University Institute of Spirituality and Health, the number of medical schools offering courses on spirituality and medicine has gone from 3 in 1992 to 72 in the year 2001.[1] But what is the nature of the spirituality that is being taught? Are all religions essentially the same, and can any spiritual leader contribute to our understanding of who God is? The exposure of spirituality in medicine is about as valid as the Christian community saying that any medicine will do.

On the positive side, various studies have shown that prayer and meditation contribute to the healing process and promote better physical, mental and emotional health. Couple that with the fact that many people in hospitals and clinics are sick for psychosomatic reasons. Surely this argues the need for wholistic health, but has this renewed interest created another monster? To what degree has Western medicine been affected by New Age and Eastern philosophies? And how has this affected Christians? The invasion of these unbiblical medical philosophies and practices into the Church may be the biggest threat to our spirituality in the twenty-first century. We routinely come across Christians who have subjected themselves to pseudomedical practices that leave them in spiritual bondage.

WESTERN MEDICINE

In addition to a serious spirituality crisis, Western medicine is also facing a financial crisis of mammoth proportions. The cost for health care and insurance is escalating beyond the average person's ability to pay. One contributing factor to the crisis is the tremendous increase in the cost of medication, which appears to be driven more by marketing than by actual necessity. For example, an Associated Press article stated, "Ask a doctor for a prescription drug you saw advertised on TV, and 69% of the time you will go home with it."[2] Julie Appleby reported in an issue of the *USA* magazine that the number of pharmaceutical representatives doubled from 41,852 in 1996 to 83,051 in the year 2000. The drug industry spent $5.3 billion in 2001 on advertising in physician journals. In the same year, more than 314,000 physician events, ranging from catered lunches in hospital rooms to getaway weekends at swank resorts, were sponsored by the drug industry. The tab was nearly $2 billion.[3]

It is not our purpose to call into question the motives of others, but this is big business and our health is at stake. That concern becomes especially evident when one considers that adverse effects from medications in hospitalized patients are so common that they are estimated to be the fourth leading cause of death in the U.S.[4] Congress has established and sets the budget for the Food and Drug Administration (FDA), which is the official sanctioning body behind prescription medication. Each year, the FDA reviews about 25 new drugs for approval. For this task, the agency has a professional staff of 1,500 doctors, scientists, toxicologists and statisticians. But to monitor the safety of the more than 3,000 drugs already on the market and being prescribed to millions, the agency has a professional staff of just five doctors and one epidemiologist.[5] Because long-term monitoring is virtually nonexistent, in a 1993 article in the *Journal of the American Medical Association*, the then commissioner of the FDA, David Kessler, revealed that "only about 1% of serious events [side effects] are reported to the FDA."[6] There is a potential risk in taking prescription medication since most side effects go unreported and nobody is sure what the long-term consequences are.

All of this has caused many to look seriously at alternative medicine. Why not give the body a chance to heal itself through good nutrition, exercise and diet? This option and possibility has often been overlooked, since the medical profession has focused primarily on illness, rather than prevention. Few medical doctors are professionally trained to offer advice on nutrition, exercise and diet. Most people would never consider going to a doctor to seek a prescription for prevention and few doctors are prepared to offer one. On the other hand, an increasing body of research shows the benefits of supplementing our diets with a balanced use of vitamins and minerals. Furthermore, the cost for nutriceuticals from health food stores is far less than the cost for pharmaceuticals, particularly when you consider the need for physician monitoring. Finally, nutriceuticals as a whole are far less toxic than prescription medication.

No wonder alternative medicine is in. But how do we know when we should take medication, when we should choose alternative medicine or when we should choose neither? Two friends with the same medical problem could be sitting side by side in the same church and hold opposite beliefs. One would first seek every possible physical explanation for their condition, with the hope that some prescription medication would cure his or her disease. The other would take medication only under extreme conditions, believing that to do so would be unwise or even a lack of faith. Which one is right?

Biblical Truth

What is lacking is true biblical integration. The problem is that when theologians have their annual meeting of the evangelical theological society, there won't be any doctors or professional counselors there. And when the American Association of Christian Counselors have their annual meeting, there won't be any doctors or theologians present. And when the Christian Medical and Dental Society convenes, there will be few—if any—theologians or psychologists present. What is needed is a national organization for Christian wholistic health where Christian theologians, doctors, nutritionists and psychologists can come together for the purpose of formulating a truly biblical basis for health.

In this book, we combine our educational and professional experiences in order to provide the reader with a grid for evaluating medical practices that are consistent with Christian beliefs. In part 1, we will examine the historical and theological roots of medicine. The goal is to provide you with a fivefold test to determine whether a medical practice or theory is wholistic and biblical. In part 2, we will look through that grid in order to evaluate medical systems. In part 3, we will evaluate several alternative therapies. In part 4, we will summarize what we have learned with a commitment to wholistic health practices that are consistent with the Word of God. Essentially, we will explain the roots of Western medicine, why it is not wholistic and why it lacks a biblical base for wholistic health. Finally, we want to acknowledge some of the benefits of alternative medicines and expose the dangers of New Age medicine.

WHOLISM VERSUS HOLISM

"Holism" is a term that was first coined by Jan Christian Smuts, a South African philosopher and statesman. In 1926, he wrote a book entitled *Holism and Evolution*, which objected to the fragmentation that viewed individuals (and the universe) as simply the sum of their parts. Smuts acknowledged the spiritual realm but seemed to perceive it more as a transcendent energy governing the whole. "Holism" all but disappeared until the 1980s, when popular New Age books revived the concept and acknowledged Smuts as the originator. While "holism" today most commonly refers to the conception of man as a functioning whole—spirit, soul and body (with which we agree)—we will continue in the Christian tradition of differentiating biblical wholism from Smuts's New Age holism by using the alternate spelling.

FINAL THOUGHTS

We don't have the final answer on theology and medicine, but God does. We encourage you to be discerning in these latter days. Whether something appears to work is not the only question we must ask. Is it right? is the ultimate question. For that we need to consult the Word of God and seek to be led by the Holy Spirit. It is our prayer that this book, with the five-point grid that you will learn in part 1, will assist you in arriving at a correct answer for the sake of your body, soul and spirit. May you prosper and be of good health, "just as your soul prospers" (3 John 2).

Neil and Michael

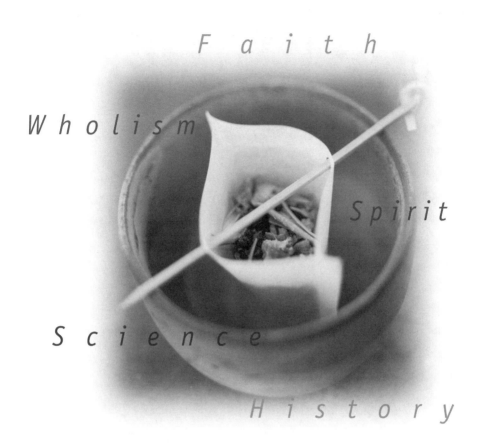

Faith

Wholism

Spirit

Science

History

PART 1

A BIBLICAL GRID FOR EVALUATING MEDICAL TREATMENTS

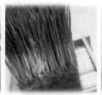

CHAPTER ONE

THE THEOLOGICAL ROOTS OF MEDICINE

The best way to show that a stick is crooked is not to argue about it nor to spend time denouncing it, but to lay a straight stick along side it.

D. L. MOODY, *THE TALE OF THE TARDY OSCART*

Many Christians believe that modern medicine is acceptable, while most everything in the alternative realm is either unproven, unscientific, quackery, a swindle or just plain devilish. While pointing out valid criticisms of alternative medical philosophies, they often do not consider the possibility that Western medicine does not necessarily equate with biblical medicine or with Christian precept. There is a simple reason for this.

The Church's primary source of health information is not taken from Scripture but comes from medical doctors trained in secular institutions with secular philosophies. When I (Michael) felt led by God to become a doctor, I didn't go to a seminary. I went to a secular medical school and was taught by professors, the majority of whom were not Christians. Furthermore, during my seven years of formal medical education, the spiritual dimension was completely ignored. Without realizing it, I was trained to divorce the physical from the spiritual. When a Christian asked me for my medical opinion, my response naturally flowed from how I was trained, which has rarely, if ever, been scrutinized by the Church.

By and large the Church has not assumed its responsibility to impact Western medicine nor evaluate what doctors are taught. When I (Neil) was preparing for the ministry, I received virtually no training in medicine or in matters relating to physical health. Not that I should have been taught the technical aspects of medicine, but I should have received some instruction on what Scripture does address. I have come to understand that the Bible has a great deal to say about how God created us in His image with a body, soul and spirit. The Bible explains why people get sick, what steps to take to prevent illness and how to get well. The Bible shows a connection between faith and healing, and teaches how diet and lifestyle affect our health. Many seminaries offer courses on medical ethics, but few teach God's perspective on health.

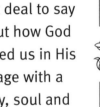

> The Bible has a great deal to say about how God created us in His image with a body, soul and spirit.

Charismatic and Pentecostal schools may emphasize miraculous healing, but they often overlook what caused the person to get ill in the first place. Consequently, church leaders conclude that when someone gets sick, they have no jurisdiction, nothing to offer, except a prayer in hope of recovery. Just like doctors, pastors have not been trained to biblically integrate the body, soul and spirit. By default, through the grid of science, doctors take care of the physical body. Pastors, through the grid of Scripture, take care of the soul and spirit.

This is terribly unfortunate, for with the inspired Word of our creator, the Church is positioned to provide excellent guidance on many of the issues that medicine is facing today. However, the Christian Church does not have a great reputation for being a strong spiritual leader in keeping medicine on the straight and narrow. Instead, in practice (not in principle) it has historically subordinated itself to whatever has been the dominant medical philosophy of the day.

HISTORY REPEATS ITSELF

For example, according to historians, for nearly 1,500 years, the Church embraced the errant teachings of Aristotle with regard to the sciences. Aristotle taught that Earth was at the center of the universe. Despite the fact that there was no scriptural requirement for such a belief, the Church held as tenaciously to this concept as it did to teachings more central to the Christian faith, such as the deity of Christ. When Galileo's observations led him to believe that the sun was at the center of the solar system, he was threatened with excommunication from the Church unless he recanted his "heretical" teaching. Scientists were thus inappropriately forced to choose between intellectual integrity and the Church. They chose the latter.[1]

Likewise, for many centuries, Greek medicine prevailed as the leading paradigm in the treatment of disease. Even to this day, Hippocrates is considered the father of modern medicine. However, this great physician accepted and practiced humoralism, an Ayurvedic/Hindu-based philosophy of medicine that emphasized the importance of balancing the body's humors (fluids). This grossly errant theory was the accepted, prevailing medical philosophy from nearly 500 B.C. until the mid-1800s! Despite the fact that its presuppositions were totally incompatible with Christian faith, the Church embraced it throughout a majority of its tenure.

> Instead of "testing the wind" and aligning itself with the prevailing medical system of our day, the Church needs to, on the basis of Scripture, establish its own philosophy and view of medicine, letting medicine align itself to it.

Today we see the same pattern. The prevailing medical philosophy in America is allopathy, and the Church has, in most respects, aligned itself with it. However, now that alternative perspectives are emerging in the medical playing field, some in the Church have joined allopathic medicine in opposing them. But for the most part, the Church is not doing so on the basis of Scripture. Even when the Church does use biblical principle as its basis for evaluation, it does not usually apply the same standard of scrutiny to allopathic medicine.

Instead of "testing the wind" and aligning itself with the prevailing medical system of our day, the Church needs to, on the basis of Scripture, establish its own philosophy and view of medicine, letting medicine align itself to it. It may seem inappropriate that the Church should involve itself in medical thinking. But far from being inappropriate, it is absolutely essential. Religious beliefs underline any system of medicine. It is religion that gives birth to philosophies in medicine. Allow us to illustrate.

MEDICAL PHILOSOPHIES EMERGE FROM RELIGION

Taoism (an ancient Eastern religion/philosophy) asserts that the first cause of the universe is immaterial energy that permeates the universe and every living being. Optimum health is only achieved when one is in harmony with the universe and when an unhindered flow of energy travels from the universe to the individual and back to the cosmos again. Therefore, all efforts to diagnose the cause of illness are oriented toward the discovery of where this energy has been blocked. In response, a variety of methods (acupuncture, acupressure, moxibustion, etc.) are utilized to remove this blockage and restore the life-giving flow. In China, Taoism gave birth to traditional Chinese medicine (see chapter 14 for a more detailed explanation of traditional Chinese medicine).

Likewise, Ayurveda, a religious system with an emphasis on maintaining balance and harmony with the universe, gave birth to humoralism (see chapter 9 for a detailed discussion). According to this theory, when illness developed, it was due to an excess of one of the body's humors. Therefore, treatment was aimed at reducing the excess, through the use of leeches, bloodletting, cathartics and so on.

Why do religious beliefs lead to medical philosophies? Because religion provides a paradigm, or blueprint, for distinguishing truth from error, right from wrong and the framework by which data is interpreted and explained. It is a worldview that attempts to provide answers to perennial human questions such as, Who am I? Why am I here? Why do people get sick and die? What is man's destiny after death? You cannot separate religious belief from medicine. Religious belief underlines not only medicine, but every other cultural institution as well, including family, education, business and government. Shared religious beliefs are essential for cohesiveness within a community and serve as the foundation for any society. Conflicting religious beliefs fracture communities as is evidenced by the continual Middle East unrest.

MEDICINE DETERIORATES OVER TIME

This concept of a connection between religion and culture and the practice of medicine is not new. Medical historians have repeatedly observed it. However, as they have researched medicine's history, they have also discovered a disturbing phenomenon that seems to appear with alarming regularity. That phenomenon has to do with what happens in medicine as a culture ages. Through examining historical records, it has become painfully evident that the best medicine that is practiced in a society is not toward the end of a particular civilization but earlier in its existence. This is exactly the opposite of what most people would expect to find. Historian Paul Ghagliounghi describes it this way:

> This was to happen over and over again in the history of medicine. Quite abruptly, pragmatic modes of medicine would emerge, which for all their limitations appear by modern standards eminently sensible, and which should have provided an excellent opportunity for a rational therapeutic system to develop. But the current would flow relentlessly the other way; rationality would be overlaid with systematization, or mumbo jumbo.[2]

But why does this deterioration in medicine occur?

> Degeneration of this kind in medical practice is usually closely related to a decline of a national culture: and so it was in Egypt. It was probably connected with the gradual falling off in regard for the gods: where a community loses faith in its traditional religion, its members are often tempted by eccentric beliefs—as if desperate for fresh certainties.[3]

As a nation or culture matures, its institutions do as well. The practice of medicine becomes systematized and great advances take place. However, at some point in time, a generation arises that questions the belief system that it has inherited. Oftentimes, this doubt is triggered by a cultural crisis such as a major military defeat, economic collapse, the ineffectiveness of religion to address the concerns of the day, or the influx of foreigners' different belief systems. In medicine, doubt can be prompted by a general realization that the current medical paradigm is ineffective in arresting common diseases.

Regardless of the reason, if a nation rejects its religious system, a crack in its foundation occurs and a cultural revolution takes place. As a result, every institution of society becomes destabilized as the nation searches for a new belief system to reestablish harmony and cohesiveness among its citizenry, and a foundation upon which to restructure its institutions. Therefore, having no unifying belief system upon which its institutions can function, the destabilized culture deteriorates, and medicine does as well.

THE CHRISTIAN CHURCH NEEDS TO SET A NEW PARADIGM

In America, the religious belief system upon which our nation was founded is Christianity. Any cursory review of original documents will confirm this. Christian precepts formed the basis for the Declaration of Independence, the Constitution and virtually every early public and private institution in America. Although, this foundation came under attack through a number of avenues, none was as dramatic as what took place in the 1960s when America endured a cultural revolution of mammoth proportions. Not surprisingly, and true to historical precedent, it was shortly thereafter that religious gurus were welcomed into the United States along with their Eastern religious teachings, such as transcendental meditation, which proliferated rapidly throughout American culture. (It seems strange that few people questioned how well those beliefs positively or negatively affected the cultures from which they came.)

During the next 30 years, Eastern concepts were gradually integrated into Western medicine. Initially, these advances were almost exclusively limited to the fringes of medical practice. However, aided by research articles showing increasing numbers of Americans flocking to these practitioners, the trickle into Western medicine rapidly became a flood. Today, doctors and medical institutions that only a few years ago banned such practices as unscientific, now embrace them with open arms and proudly practice them. Evidence that this major ideological shift has taken place abounds throughout the health-care system.

1. Like many other cities, virtually every major hospital system in Cincinnati has built a health and fitness center where patients are encouraged to partake in classes ranging from acupuncture to qigong to reflexology to yoga. What a dramatic shift from just a few years ago when all of these practices were considered unscientific, if not outright quackery.

2. In the last few years, numerous continuing medical education (CME) brochures from Harvard Medical School have touted keynote

speakers who have been invited to address issues of spirituality, usually from an Eastern mysticism perspective. Harvard, once the icon of the purely biochemical, scientific medical model, now hosts conferences on spirituality and healing in conjunction with the Mind/Body Medical Institute at Beth Israel Deaconess Medical Center.

3. Required physician CME conferences commonly include lectures on spirituality and alternative medicine. Recently such an event in Vermont featured a lecture on spirituality. During the question and answer period that followed, attendees were given a brochure inviting them to a retreat in the North Carolina mountains. This weekend event was designed to help physicians rediscover "the archetypal energy of the healer" that first led them to practice medicine and to experience a "re-animation" of "the healer within." Speakers included a psychotherapist who specialized in understanding the relationship between symptoms and intrapersonal energies of the soul. Another therapist had extensive experience with various shaman healers and rituals. And native American counselors guided participants on their journey of "longing toward healing for ourselves and for the whole of creation."[4]

So where does that leave us? Western medicine (and our society), in the wake of a cultural revolution, is in a state of flux and confusion as it searches for a unifying belief system. Consistent with historical precedent, the paths in this search for truth have led to Eastern belief systems. Meanwhile, the Church has been hampered in its ability to be a reconciling force because it has blindly accepted Western allopathic medicine as being consistent with Christian belief. This is despite the fact that the philosophical underpinnings of allopathic medicine have, for most of its history, been rooted in a pagan belief system contrary to Christianity.

Since the ultimate cause of our present crisis has to do with foundational religious beliefs, the solution must be found at that level. America has a Christian heritage. The Church, in many respects, is still looked to as a reference point, particularly in regard to truth. This is a golden opportunity for the Church, perhaps one that has not been available for a long time. Medicine and society at large are grasping for a unifying worldview that combines faith with real life and provides answers not only to the larger questions in life but also a legitimate framework for medical decision making in the face of illness.

The Church must come forth with a paradigm for medicine that is consistent with biblical faith and is compatible with legitimate science. Christian patients and physicians are in desperate need for a reconnection between biblical faith, physical health and medical practice. For that matter, so is the rest of the world.

CHAPTER TWO

THE NEED FOR A COMPREHENSIVE MEANS OF EVALUATION

Christianity is not a drug that suits some complaints and not others.
It is either sheer illusion or else it is the Truth. But if it is the Truth, if the
universe happens to be constituted in this way, the question is not whether
the God of Christianity suits us, but whether we suit Him.

WILLIAM TEMPLE

THE CASE IN QUESTION

Ralph and Amy were dear friends. A vivacious 69-year-old Christian, Amy had enjoyed excellent health throughout most of her life. Now she found herself engaged in a desperate struggle to regain her health. Ralph and Amy asked me, "Would you go with us to Amy's next appointment and give your input?" I (Michael) wanted to do anything I could to help them out of their predicament, so I agreed to go.

A Devastating Illness

Several months earlier, doctors had discovered that Amy's blood pressure was out of control. On any given day, she could easily drive the mercury to over 200/120, hard to imagine in such a petite woman who barely broke the five-foot barrier.

Ever since her diagnosis, she had tried to rein in the hypertension on her own by going "natural." A strict vegetarian when her illness began, she at first tried juices, supplements and finally herbs. Even though she was a retired nurse, she loathed the idea of taking medications. To her, drugs were equivalent to poison.

But eventually the poison won out; her disease got the best of her. She suffered a series of devastating strokes. In response, her doctors put her on digoxin to control her abnormal heartbeat, warfarin to keep her blood from clotting (this actually is an ingredient of rat poison) and a series of various high-blood-pressure medications, none of which were effective.

Still looking for a better answer, a Christian friend recommended a local chiropractor. This doctor was not only reported to be a Christian, but he was also very oriented toward finding the root cause of health problems and treating them with diets, herbs and supplements. All this had sounded very appealing to Ralph and Amy, since it seemed that this doctor thought very similarly to how they did with regard to obtaining optimum health.

Amy went to her first appointment two weeks before our scheduled appointment together. While there, she became quite impressed with this young doctor, although she was a little puzzled by his approach. It certainly was very different from what she had seen during her nursing days. Having heard me (Michael) lecture on the benefits and potential pitfalls of alternative medicine, Amy and Ralph approached me to see if I would be interested in helping them evaluate this medical philosophy by accompanying them to her follow-up appointment. I decided to accept their invitation and found it to be a very interesting experience.

The Office Visit

After being seated in the waiting room for a few minutes, a nurse called us back to a rear treatment room. In addition to a few chairs and a desk, it contained several bookshelves of supplements and a novel computer arrangement. Connected to the computer's central processor was a 12-inch square metal tray with two wires attached at opposite corners. Exiting one corner was a wire with a red (positive) electrode, which Amy was asked to hold in her right hand. At the opposite corner was another wire attached to a black (negative) electrode. This sensor was held in the right hand of the chiropractor.

Taking Amy's left hand into his, the chiropractor touched specific points on her hand with the negative electrode. "These points," he explained, "correspond with specific organ systems or disease processes within the body. Every organ in the body and every disease have a specific frequency associated with it. We can test for each of these frequencies and assess the status of each particular system. If the system is healthy, a proper amount of energy will be flowing through it."

As he touched each point, the computer graphed a blue bar across the screen, representing the energy present in that particular organ or system. If the system was healthy, the computer verified this by plotting a blue bar graph that stopped midway on the screen. However, if there was a problem, the bar graph either fell short of the midline (too little energy) or went clear across the screen (too much energy).

In this way, each system in the body was tested and a list of problem areas was developed. Then for each problem area, a bottled supplement or herb was selected from the shelves and placed into the middle of the metal tray. Problem areas were retested with the energy now passing through the patient and then through the remedy before reaching the computer. If the remedy was helpful, it would cause one or more of the problem bar graphs to become balanced in the middle of the screen. Those remedies that were deemed helpful were then set aside. After individual testing was complete, the entire regimen, consisting of approximately one dozen bottles, was placed in the center of the metal tray and retested altogether.

The final step was to determine the correct dosage for each remedy. This was accomplished by having Amy take each remedy individually into her right hand. While holding it close to her chest, the chiropractor tested the muscle strength of her outstretched left arm. With each item tested, he turned to his assistant and said, "She needs two of these each day" or "She needs four of these." The most he prescribed of any one remedy was six.

Having completed his assessment, the young doctor kindly thanked us for coming, shook our hands and exited the room. I then asked his assistant how he was able to tell how much of the remedy to prescribe to his patient. "Oh, that's easy," she replied. "He just asked her body, and her body told him." I had been standing a matter of inches away from this doctor, yet I had not heard him ask her for this information. Obviously, it was something that he had ascertained without uttering words out loud.

The Doctor's Regimen

The appointment was brought to a close as the entire regimen was written up on paper and given to Amy. As we walked out into the parking lot, Ralph and

Amy turned to me and asked, "So what do you think? Does it look good? Is everything okay?"

What would you tell Ralph and Amy? Are they going down the right path? And upon what basis would you formulate your answer? Most important, would God be able to use you to give wise counsel to these children of His who are looking to you for direction?

THE NEED FOR AN EVALUATIVE PROCESS CONSISTENT WITH SCRIPTURE

On the West Bank of the Potomac River in Arlington, Virginia, stands the Pentagon, one of the great architectural achievements of the twentieth century. Since 1943, this nearly 4-million-square-foot building has been home to the United States Department of Defense. Perhaps most unique to this stately structure is its design that repeats itself in multiples of five. Having five sides and a mile-long perimeter, it also has five stories and five concentric rings. Over the years, the Pentagon has become for many a symbol of strength, stability and protection. Although terrorists tried to bring it down, it still stands.

> What is needed in addressing the medical issues of our day is a reliable and enduring biblical model that will stand the test of time.

What is needed in addressing the medical issues of our day is a reliable and enduring biblical model that will stand the test of time. Like the Pentagon, our method of evaluation will be constructed with five sides, or perspectives, by which we will examine various medical philosophies and practices. No one perspective in and of itself offers a complete view. All five sides are needed in order to provide a 360-degree look. Over the next several chapters, this five-dimensional grid, which we have developed in a manner fully consistent with Scripture, will be explained in greater detail. Once the grid is established, we will then evaluate a number of common medical philosophies including modern Western medicine, using the five-dimensional grid. Summarized briefly, the five grids are as follows:

1. The grid of **history**—The first step in looking at a medical philosophy is to look at its historical roots. Who invented it and how was it developed? This information will shed light on each of the remaining issues.

2. The grid of **faith**—As we explained in chapter 1, every medical system flows from a foundation of religious beliefs. Using the Bible as our standard of reference, how do the spiritual concepts underlying the founder and medical system in question line up? Are they consistent with biblical precept and historical Christian faith?

3. The **wholistic** grid—Does the medical philosophy properly address the whole person (spirit, soul and body) or just one dimension? Any medical system that discounts or disregards one or more of these components of humanity may be effective in one dimension, but it will have significant limitations in its usefulness on a broader scale.

4. The grid of **science**—How does the approach in question line up with natural law? Nature is governed by fixed, universal principles that cannot be violated without consequence. Does this medical philosophy work consistently with known natural law, to the best of our understanding?

5. The grid of **spiritual discernment**—Scripture warns us, "Beloved, believe not every spirit, but try the spirits whether they are of God: because many false prophets are gone out into the world" (1 John 4:1, *KJV*). The Holy Spirit is the Spirit of truth, and He will lead you into all truth. The devil is the father of lies and his demons will make every attempt to deceive you. This is a critical issue since the apostle Paul warned the Church, "The Spirit clearly says that in later times some will abandon the faith and follow deceiving spirits and things taught by demons" (1 Tim. 4:1, *NIV*).

These five grids serve as a practical guide in determining God's direction for medical decision making, particularly in regard to the type of care, or approach, one is considering. However, nothing supersedes the personal guidance of the Holy Spirit in an individual's life. Jesus comments on the Holy Spirit:

Nevertheless I tell you the truth; it is expedient for you that I go away: for if I go not away, the Comforter will not come unto you; but if

I depart, I will send him unto you. Howbeit when he, the Spirit of truth, is come, he will guide you into all truth" (John 16:7,13, *KJV*).

Jesus could have stuck around forever after His resurrection. He had a new body—He was immortal. Just think: if He was around, we could call Him up and ask Him what we need to know. But that wasn't God's plan. It's not that Jesus did not want to be around us. He had something better. He came to give us eternal spiritual life and by doing so He would dwell within us. Jesus wanted to commune with all of us in a personal way. As children of God, our souls are in union with God. Every born-again believer is alive and free in Christ. He left this earth in order that He might indwell us through the person of the Holy Spirit.

> God has the only perfect perspective on an individual's needs, and He has promised to lead us into all truth.

With this in mind, let us return to Amy and Ralph's case. The most important question that needs to be asked is, How is the Holy Spirit leading Ralph and Amy? Each person is unique and every treatment is not necessarily right for every individual. There are some people who can eat one peanut and die, while others enjoy this wonderful provision without a care. Paul wrote, "All things are lawful, but not all things are profitable. All things are lawful, but not all things edify" (1 Cor. 10:23). In other words, what God has created for food and provision is lawful, but it may not always be the best for you. God has the only perfect perspective on an individual's needs, and He has promised to lead us into all truth. It is possible that the first four grids might check out okay, but that does not necessarily mean God is directing Amy to pursue that particular medical regimen. Conversely, the treatment approach may not perfectly line up with the first four grids, but it is possible that the Holy Spirit may still direct an individual to utilize it. The fifth test—spiritual discernment—is the only one that must always be passed. If a spirit is involved and it is not the Holy Spirit, then there is no way that the Holy Spirit will sanction it. As we work through the next five chapters, we will use Amy's case scenario to show how to address her question through each of the five grids.

With a little historical background (there wasn't much!) on the doctor's system and its development (the first grid), and the religious system upon which it was based (the second grid), Ralph and Amy realized that the doctor's wholistic approach (the third grid) was not compatible with a biblical view of man. Furthermore, we were able to find only a few instances in which this system had been scientifically tested and these studies conflicted with one another; therefore, it failed the grid of science (the fourth grid). Finally, in looking through the grid of spiritual discernment (the fifth grid), at least one aspect of Amy's evaluation bore significant resemblance to practices used in divination. As a result, Ralph and Amy determined that despite the fact that this practitioner supposedly professed Christianity in his personal life, his professional approach appeared incompatible with biblical faith.

FINAL THOUGHTS

Several key issues need to be addressed before we expand upon these five grids. You will soon notice that there is no single medical approach that lines up perfectly with every test. Every system of medicine that we have examined falls short in some way, including our Western scientific system. This implies several things:

1. There is a great need for dialogue between the Church and the medical profession. While every medical system traces its heritage to religious parentage, there is no medical system (that we have found) that can truly claim Christianity as its birthright, yet Christians believe that the Bible holds the answers to questions that directly impinge upon life, death and health. Pastors, Christian leaders, health-care educators and providers need to dialogue with one another.

2. We hope to avoid making the same mistake that the Church has made in previous generations. That is, we want to avoid automatically aligning ourselves with any prevailing medical model simply because it is regulated by the government and sanctioned by leading medical institutions. As you will learn in chapter 10, the only pillar supporting Western allopathic medicine is science (and even that is not always the case). We must be honest in identifying what each medical philosophy is consistent with and where each is contrary to biblical precept.

3. If you are sick and need to see a doctor, you will probably utilize the services of a health-care provider and a system that is not in complete

agreement with your faith. It is not our intention to discredit every doctor nor do we want you to decline help that is available simply because it does not pass all the tests. If you did that, you would be left without any service at all.

4. Particularly in the field of medicine, you cannot sacrifice professional competency for the sake of spiritual agreement. A bright Christian doctor could subscribe to everything we say, but he or she would be a poor choice if he or she has poor medical skills. Dedicated incompetence is still incompetence. If you are planning triple bypass surgery, it is probably better to select a pagan veteran of many successful surgeries than to have a young Christian doctor perform his or her first open-heart surgery on you. However, you may consider asking him or her to assist and pray for you.

5. No one doctor is going to be perfectly wholistic. Establishing Christian wholistic health is going to require all the disciplines of body, soul and mind to come together under the umbrella of Scripture in order to address the needs of the whole person. Your wholistic experience will probably be made complete through Christian friends, church, pastoral counseling or Christ-centered therapy, and sound teaching on health that assists you in developing a prudent lifestyle.

6. As you will learn in chapter 4, a person's lifestyle can be the source for all kinds of diseases and illnesses. There are no promises in the Bible that say we don't have to live with the physical consequences of a sinful life. Languishing in bitterness and self-inflicted stress will have a negative impact on our health. Perhaps you abused alcohol. While God will forgive your chemical abuse, you may still have to live with cirrhosis of the liver.

7. Unless Christ returns first, you're going to have to die of something. God's Word is good preventative medicine; it is also healing. You can make the choice right now to live a righteous life and make the commitment to live by faith in the power of the Holy Spirit according to what God said is true. But you are still living in a fallen world and residing in a decaying body. Even if you lived perfectly according to Scripture, your body will still fail somewhere in order for death to come. The purpose for living a righteous life is to glorify

God, to walk in fellowship with Him and to be a good steward of what He has entrusted to you. Maintaining a Christ-centered focus while living a balanced, prudent life with proper exercise and diet are central to good stewardship. Optimum physical health flows from these priorities.

We hope that the concepts presented in this book will enable you to keep your faith in Christ and discern God's direction while you navigate through the maze of medicine.

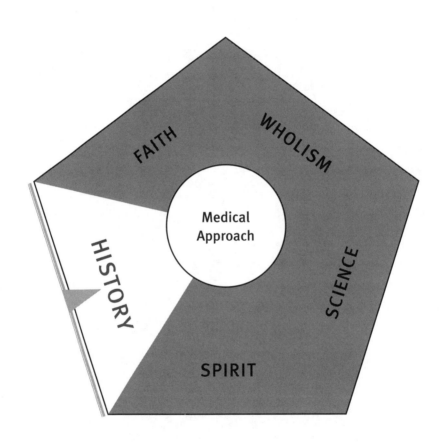

CHAPTER THREE

EVALUATING THROUGH THE GRID OF HISTORY

Those who don't know history are forever condemned to repeat it.

WILL DURANT

The first step in biblically testing a medical philosophy is to look at its history. Where did the system of medicine originate? Who was its founder? What information do we know about his or her life and teachings? What were his or her religious beliefs? What was the basis for their faith and what did they believe about the cause and cure of illnesses? While this first step is not a literal test, the information gleaned from it is valuable to evaluating the philosophy through the remaining four grids.

Since what we are most interested in is an understanding of a Christian view of health, healing and medicine, this chapter will principally focus on the biblical history of health care as well as the Christian history of health care that followed the close of the writing of the Scriptures.

A BIBLICAL PERSPECTIVE ON MODERN MEDICINE

At first glance, it would appear that biblical Christianity and medicine have very little in common with one another. No hospitals or clinics are mentioned in the Bible, and there are very few places where we find the words "medicine" or "physician." Of those that do occur, they serve to be quite humbling to those of us in this healing profession. The first occurrence of the word "physician" is found in Genesis 50:2 ("physicians"), where we discover that Egyptian doctors were responsible for embalming dead people. The next reference involves King Asa who was criticized because he only sought the counsel of physicians and did not seek the Lord (see 2 Chron. 16:12). The implication is that his mistake cost him his life. Another reference is when Job referred to his friends as "physicians of no value" (Job 13:4, *KJV*).

In his gospel, Mark records an incident in which a woman who had a bleeding disorder for 12 years merely touched Jesus' clothes and was healed. According to the apostle, this woman "had endured much at the hands of many physicians, and had spent all that she had and was not helped at all, but rather had grown worse" (Mark 5:26). The same event was also recorded by Luke, "the beloved physician" (Col. 4:14) who was apparently beloved, not for his medical expertise, but because of his faithfulness to Christ and the apostle Paul. Nothing is written as to his practice of medicine.

Why does it appear that medicine and physicians were held in such low esteem? The first answer seems obvious. Certainly the medicine of 2,000 years ago was largely ineffective. The need for sterility was not common knowledge; therefore, surgery carried with it a high mortality rate. For 500 years before Christ and for 1,800 years after, Greek humoralism dominated the medical landscape. As we will learn in chapter 10, this philosophy was rooted in a pagan belief system and was characterized by harsh treatments such as purgatives, emetics and toxic drugs. This is probably the type of medicine in which Luke was trained.

But beyond medicine's apparent ineffectiveness, there stands a greater reason why there is so little mention of medicine in Scripture. The Hebrews had a very clearly defined worldview, and not one of the prevailing medical systems was compatible with it. The children of Israel understood that God was their creator and that disease and death came into the world as a direct result of sin. Moses told them that if they walked in righteousness as a nation, God would protect them from disease (see Exod. 15:26); but if they forsook God, His protective blessing would be removed and the nation would be cursed. Secular physicians were unlikely to consider these concepts when treating their patients. Their practices were rooted in pagan belief systems and often closely tied with occult activities, including idol worship, which made procurement of their services tantamount to consulting with a sorcerer.

THE INFLUENCE OF CHRIST

By the time of Christ, Israel showed great evidence that she was an apostate nation under the curse of the law. Everywhere one looked there was disease. Deafness and blindness were commonplace, as were instances of obvious demonization. The Gospels are replete with references to those who were disfigured, paralyzed or plagued with leprosy, the diagnosis of which inevitably resulted in a curse of uncleanness and ostracism from the community.

Into this vast sea of human suffering and need came the God-man who would alter the course of history and change the face of humanity forever. He had the authority to forgive sins and unlimited power to heal disease. Matthew wrote that "great multitudes came" to Jesus, bringing "with them those that were lame, blind, dumb, maimed, and many others" (Matt. 15:30, *KJV*). Jesus healed them and the multitudes witnessed "the dumb to speak, the maimed to be whole, the lame to walk, and the blind to see" (v. 31, *KJV*). Consequently, "they glorified the God of Israel" (v. 31, *KJV*). Luke, a trained doctor, must have been in awe when he penned these words about the great physician.

> Now when the sun was setting, all they that had any sick with divers diseases brought them unto him; and he laid his hands on every one of them, and healed them. And devils also came out of many, crying out, and saying, Thou art Christ the Son of God. And he rebuking them suffered them not to speak: for they knew that he was Christ (Luke 4:40-41, *KJV*).

Matthew explained that Jesus' ability to "cast out the spirits with a word" and heal "all who were ill" was confirmation that He was the promised Messiah (Matt. 8:16-17), fulfilling that which was spoken by Isaiah the prophet, who said that Jesus "took up our infirmities and carried our sorrows" (Isa. 53:4).

Secular historians do not usually deny the accounts of Jesus' miraculous healings. However, some try to explain them away, saying that sick people were made well by Jesus' power of suggestion.[1] That seems hardly feasible. How does the power of suggestion account for someone who has been paralyzed since birth? Did no one before Jesus ever think to tell the paralytic to just get up? And how could the power of suggestion raise Lazarus from the grave, someone who had been dead in a tomb for four days. According to his sister, "by this time he stinketh" (John 11:39, KJV). Some have suggested that Jesus had to call Lazarus by name or all of the dead would have come forth (see John 11:1-45)!

No, it is obvious that Jesus had much more than the power of suggestion. He had an awesome power to heal and even raise people from the dead.

THE POWER TO HEAL

During Jesus' earthly ministry, he not only healed but also extended His power and authority to His disciples and told them to use it to heal the sick and free the oppressed.

> And when he had called unto him his twelve disciples, he gave them power against unclean spirits, to cast them out, and to heal all manner of sickness and all manner of disease. Heal the sick, cleanse the lepers, raise the dead, cast out devils: freely ye have received, freely give (Matt. 10:1,8, KJV).

This power was also evident in the lives of the disciples after Jesus had ascended into heaven and after they had received the Holy Spirit at Pentecost.

> And by the hands of the apostles were many signs and wonders wrought among the people. Insomuch that they brought forth the sick into the streets, and laid them on beds and couches, that at the least the shadow of Peter passing by might overshadow some of them. There came also a multitude out of the cities round about unto Jerusalem, bringing sick folks, and them which were vexed with unclean spirits: and they were healed every one (Acts 5:12, 15-16, KJV).

In Galatia, Paul healed a man who had been crippled from birth (see Acts 14:8-10). In Philippi, he cast out a spirit of divination (see Acts 16:16-18), and in Ephesus "God wrought special miracles by the hands of Paul" so that the sick were healed by even his handkerchief (Acts 19:11-12, KJV). On his trip to Rome, his prayerful laying on of hands healed the father of Publius (see Acts 28:8).

Peter and Paul were also each used by God to raise two people from the dead (see Acts 9:36-41; 20:9-12).

Theologians have noticed that the occurrence of miracles and healing begins to diminish in the book of Acts as the Church matured and spread. Miraculous physical healings were not emphasized in Early Church historical writings, and it appears that the Church did not continue facilitating the miraculous intervention of Christ in the lives of His children, including supernatural healing. (For further discussion on where the miracles of healing are today, see appendix A.)

THE COMPASSION TO CARE

After the Apostolic Age, the Church largely turned its attention away from miracles to caring for the sick. This also was in keeping with the example of Christ, who demonstrated limitless compassion for those who were suffering. His capacity to love has not been overlooked by secular historians. Brian Inglis, who to our knowledge never claimed to be a follower of Christ, asserted that no other historical figure had a greater impact on the delivery of health care than Jesus. The reason for his proposal was the extraordinary compassion that Jesus Christ demonstrated for the sick and the poor. According to Inglis, no prophet of any other religion bore this quality.[2]

That same spirit of compassion was passed on to Jesus' followers to such an extent that the Early Church is credited with establishing the first hospitals. The love and concern that these Christians had for the sick was so profound that it was perceived as a major threat to the Roman empire. In the fourth century, Emperor Julian the Apostate complained:

> Now we can see what it is that makes these Christians such powerful
> enemies of our gods; it is the brotherly love that they manifest toward
> strangers, the sick and the poor.[3]

Despite the fact that Western medicine has now become big business, evidence of this Christian legacy of love still permeates our nation's health-care system as many hospitals still retain the names of the denominations that founded them.

However, while the hearts of many rendering care to the sick have borne Christ's spirit of compassion throughout the centuries, the philosophies upon which that medical care is based have historically not been consistent with His teachings. As healing miracles faded with the close of the Apostolic Age, Christians caring for the sick resorted to contemporary medical philosophies and practices to diagnose and treat illness. This is still true today. I (Michael) wrote in chapter 1 how that when I felt God call me into medicine, I went to a medical school where I was trained in a secular system that not only fails to consider biblical revelation but also is often antagonistic to it. Therefore, as I cared for the sick, I may have done so with a heart of compassion, much like that of our Lord Jesus, but my mind was filled with the ideas of men. Now some of those ideas appear to be good and right, but in the light of Scripture, others clearly fall short.

THE AUTHORITATIVE SOURCE FOR FAITH AND PRACTICE

That is not to say that all a Christian physician needs to do is study the Scriptures in order to fully understand how to practice medicine. Although the Bible is the sole authority for our faith and worldview, it is not a text that medical doctors would use to diagnose and treat diseases (particularly those with a physical root cause), set broken legs or transplant organs. God has left humanity with a large share of the responsibility for discovering what He has created.

For example, in Leviticus we find helpful information in regard to leprosy. But while some details were provided to the Hebrews as to how to make the diagnosis of this dreaded disease, no treatment was prescribed other than isolation from those who weren't afflicted. Several thousand years later, researchers discovered that leprosy is caused by a bacterium (*Mycobacterium leprae*) that attacks the nerves.[4] When Jesus walked the face of the earth, He cured many people who were blind. Then why didn't He explain the principles of optics so that everybody with poor vision could just get corrective lenses?

Proverbs 25:2 (*KJV*) says, "It is the glory of God to conceal a thing: but the honour of kings is to search out a matter." God gave Adam and Eve the mandate to "be fruitful and multiply, and fill the earth, and subdue it; and rule over the fish of the sea and over the birds of the sky, and over every living thing that moves on the earth" (Gen. 1:28). Adam, Eve and their descendants were given the responsibility to study creation and to learn its secrets. However, this was not to be accomplished independently of God. The Lord will provide the guidance we need and enable the process if we stay in an intimate relationship with Him.

Like society in general, many Christian health-care professionals are searching for a unifying worldview that acknowledges the reality of the spiritual world. They believe in biblical revelation but see a disconnection between their faith and the practice of scientific medicine. They need a wholistic medical paradigm that integrates biblical faith with legitimate medical science. On the other hand, the Church is in need of a medical paradigm that is consistent with what they know to be true—the holy Scriptures. As we will see in the next chapters, Christianity offers the foundation upon which such a medical paradigm can and should be built.

> **The Church is in need of a medical paradigm that is consistent with what they know to be true—the holy Scriptures.**

RALPH AND AMY'S APPLICATION #1

The first step in evaluating a medical approach is to look at it its history. Usually, the place to start is with the practitioner. I (Michael) asked Amy's chiropractor (see story in chapter 2) the following questions. His answers (paraphrased by me) are italicized.

1. What is the name of the approach that you are using and where did it originate? *It is known as electrodermal testing. It used to be called EAV, which stands for electrodiagnosis according to Voll. In the 1930s, Reinhold Voll discovered that he could measure skin resistance at acupuncture points, which provided an objective measurement of the energy status of corresponding meridians and their respective organ systems. Various devices have been invented for that purpose, including the Vegatest. About 14 years ago, the computerized system that I use was developed.* [The muscle-testing technique that Amy's chiropractor used was a variation of applied kinesiology (AK), which, as you will learn in chapter 16, was developed by a Detroit-area chiropractor named George Goodheart.]

2. How did you learn of it? *I heard of it several years ago and traveled to Germany where I was trained in its use by Helmut Schimmel.*

3. Why is it not used by more physicians? *A variety of practitioners in the U.S. are using it; however, it has not gained wide acceptance. There is no CPT (billing code) for it (i.e., it is not recognized as a legitimate treatment by insurance companies), and some medical licensing boards are antagonistic to it. For example, a Florida physician lost his license for using electrodermal testing in his practice.*

This sampling of questions about the history and development of the system should give you an idea of the kinds of questions you should ask. With the historical information in hand, you might next consult a Christian reference book (such as parts 2 and 3 of this book) or a secular work. Regarding the latter, be aware of the fact that a majority of secular books on alternative medicine endorse a variety of practices that are potentially objectionable to the Christian faith. Nevertheless, we have found them helpful resources in providing us raw data or information; however, we have not sought them for their opinions. As we proceed through the remaining four grids, additional information will shed further light on Amy's question, "Is everything okay with this practitioner's medical approach?"

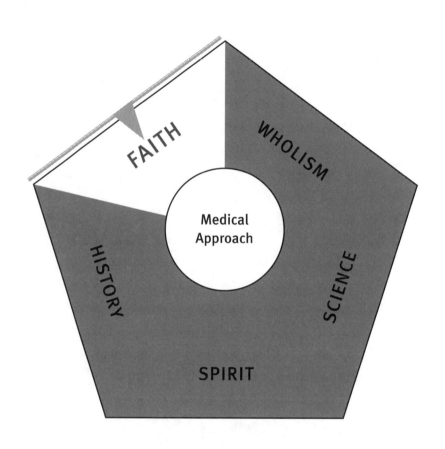

CHAPTER FOUR

EVALUATING THROUGH THE GRID OF FAITH

Faith . . . is a steady and certain knowledge of the Divine benevolence towards us, which, being founded on the truth and the gratuitous promise of Christ, is both revealed to our minds, and confirmed in our hearts, by the Holy Spirit.

JOHN CALVIN, *INSTITUTES OF THE CHRISTIAN RELIGION*

The second step in evaluating a medical system is to identify the religion upon which that system is based. As was set forth in chapter 1, every medical philosophy flows from a system of religious belief. Are the basic tenets of the medical solution that you are considering consistent with those of Christianity? In order to evaluate this, we must first have a clear understanding of those principles that are central to the Christian faith.

THE AUTHORITY OF SCRIPTURE

Every established religion looks to an authoritative teacher as the founder of its religion and to a canon of writings as the basis for its doctrine, teaching, government and function. For Islam, it is Mohammed and the Koran. For Judaism, it is the Old Testament, which contains the writings of the ancient patriarchs and prophets, and the Talmud, with its rabbinical interpretation. The Old Testament is a historical account of creation, the Fall and God's unfolding plan for redemption. Moses, the lawgiver, revealed the holiness of God and provided instructions for living a righteous life under the Law. The problem was nobody could live a righteous life by the Law. The Law was a taskmaster to lead us to Christ.

Christianity acknowledges the Old Testament as being authoritative, believing that its prophetic claims of a messianic deliverer are fulfilled in the person of Jesus Christ. Christ came to resolve the enmity that existed between fallen humanity and God. He did so by dying for our sins, and then He gave us eternal spiritual life. His death also undid the works of Satan. Then after the death and resurrection of Jesus, the Holy Spirit came upon every believer to be once again united to God in Christ. Being alive in Christ means that our souls are in union with God:

> He who raised Christ Jesus from the dead will also *give life to your mortal bodies* through His Spirit who indwells you (Rom. 8:11, emphasis added).

Religion is by nature exclusive. All religious systems (even atheism and humanism) claim to profess the truth. Therefore, any teaching that is contrary to that belief system is assumed to be false. This concept is an excessively large pill to swallow for many in our pluralistic society. However, we all live by this principle every day.

In baseball, a hit down the line is either ruled a foul ball or a fair ball—it can't be both. In math, two plus two equals four—no other number is an acceptable answer. A traffic light must give one signal—a double message would result in chaos. Medicine also, by nature, is exclusive—either the individual has a particular disease, or he or she does not. If someone is told that they have tuberculosis when in fact their problem is lung cancer, the diagnosis is wrong. I (Neil) struggled for nine months with what doctors diagnosed as bronchitis. It only got worse until I checked into emergency care and doctors put me on oxygen. Finally, it was discovered that I had exercise-induced asthma. The truth led to the right diagnosis and treatment.

It is the truth of divine revelation that is the plumb line for evaluating all other religions.

It is the truth of divine revelation that is the plumb line for evaluating all other religions. Therefore, it is imperative that we understand clearly what our faith proclaims: What is the Christian view of humanity, and why do we get sick, and how do we get well? Answers to these questions are essential to determining a Christian perspective on medicine. While some of the following concepts may seem very basic, many directly contradict the medical philosophies of today.

THE BASICS OF CHRISTIANITY

God, Man and Creation

The Scriptures teach that in the beginning was God (see Gen. 1:1), a living Spirit who preceded all physical matter. God created Adam and Eve in His own image, a physical representation of His likeness. They were to tend the garden and rule over all other creation (see Gen. 1:26-27). As a result, man has been given special and unique value amongst all creation. Yet, man is separate and inferior from his creator. By virtue of the fact that God created man and gave him life, He has a divine right over His creation.

Jesus clearly demonstrated His superiority over both the physical and the spiritual realm. According to Genesis 1:31, everything that God made "was very good"—it was perfect. Originally, man had a wonderful, untarnished and mutually loving relationship with his creator. God used to walk in the cool of the day with Adam and Eve (see Gen. 3:8). Life and fellowship with God was immediate and continuous. Adam and Eve also had a perfect, harmonious and loving relationship with one another. They were naked and unashamed. They never considered any part of their body to be dirty, and there was nothing immoral about sex. There was no disease or death. In fact, the Scriptures imply that man was originally designed to live forever.

Evil

The flawless utopia was soon marred by the appearance of evil, which, from man's perspective, first manifested itself in the form of a serpent (see Gen. 3:1). Prior to creation as we know it, Satan was not created evil. According to the prophets Ezekiel and Isaiah, he was God's highest created being. As an angel who led heaven's worship, Satan was endowed with awesome beauty and power. But having a subordinate role eventually became unacceptable to him.

Corrupted by an unquenchable thirst for power and equality with God, he was cast out of heaven. Along with him were expelled one-third of the host-of-heaven angels, who had also become tainted with the same rebellious attitude (see Isa. 14:12-15).

The evil one is referred to throughout Scripture by a variety of descriptive names, including Lucifer (from "lucent" or "light," alluding to his former glory in heaven), Satan (which means "to attack"), the adversary, the father of lies, the great deceiver and the devil. Since his removal from heaven, Satan has continued his efforts at establishing his earthly kingdom apart from the rule and reign of God. His kingdom was initially comprised of angelic beings that joined him in his rebellion. Referred to as demons, these "fallen angels" continuously oppose God and attempt to corrupt all that is righteous and holy.

Before long he directed those efforts toward mankind. Through deception and lies, the adversary seduced man into disobeying God, thereby fracturing the holy, pure and life-giving relationship that man had enjoyed with his creator (see Gen. 3). The results of man's disobedience were disastrous—disease and death were now part of man's being (see Gen. 2:17). Satan usurped the dominion that God intended for Adam and His descendants. He became the rebel holder of authority, "the ruler of this world" (John 16:11) and "the prince of the power of the air" (Eph. 2:2, *KJV*). Consequently, "the whole world lies in the power of the evil one . . . who deceives the whole world" (1 John 5:19; Rev. 12:9).

> The god of this world has blinded the minds of the unbelieving, that they might not see the light of the gospel of the glory of Christ, who is the image of God (2 Cor. 4:4).

Should Satan lose the battle for our souls, and we turn to Christ for salvation, he doesn't just give up his efforts to undermine our lives. He still tempts us to live independent of God, accuses us of all our sins and deceives us into believing his lies. He can't do anything about our position in Christ, but if he can get us to believe it isn't true, we will live as though it isn't.

It is critical to understand Satan's evil attacks on our physical and mental health for two reasons. First, the primary battle is for the mind. If we believe the father of lies, we will not live righteously according to God's perfect plan for us. Believing the father of lies can lead to all kinds of psychosomatic illnesses. Second, Satan apparently has some ability to affect us physically. Most of this is also centered in the mind. For instance, after Christ set the demonized man free, he was "in his right mind" (Mark 5:15, *KJV*). Over 25 percent of the physical healings in the Gospel of Mark were the result of Jesus expelling demons. Luke records the story of "a woman who for eighteen years had had a sickness caused by a spirit; and she was bent double, and could not straighten up" (Luke 13:11). It would be easy in our Western world to see only the physical effects and not the cause of this woman's sickness today. Jesus made it clear that this "daughter of Abraham" was bound by Satan (see Luke 13:16, *KJV*). Obviously not all illnesses are satanically induced, but Scripture teaches that some may be.

Disease and Death

When Adam sinned, he died spiritually and lost the inherent capacity to fellowship with his creator. Since then, every descendant of Adam and Eve has been born physically alive but spiritually dead (see Eph. 2:1). Because of this estrangement from God, we have lost the ability to accurately comprehend spiritual things.

> But the natural man receiveth not the things of the Spirit of God: for they are foolishness unto him: neither can he know them, because they are spiritually discerned (1 Cor. 2:14, *KJV*).

However, God provides us with a plan of redemption, which gives us the opportunity to be "born again" (John 3:3). And when we receive Christ, we "become children of God" (John 1:12, *NKJV*). We receive the mind of Christ (see 1 Cor. 2:16) and the indwelling of the Holy Spirit, which leads us into all truth (see John 16:13). "All truth" includes instruction for righteous living, as well as how to live in such a way that ensures better physical and mental health.

Paul challenges believers not to be deceived by pagan practices that exclude Christ and divine revelation.

> See to it that no one takes you captive through philosophy and empty deception . . . according to the elementary principles of the world, rather than according to Christ (Col. 2:8).

Deceptive philosophies and practices include humanistic medicine that treats only the body and sees only science as the standard for faith. It also includes secular psychology that possesses no biblical understanding of God and what it means to be a child of God.

Adam and Eve's rebellion brought disease, death and a corruption of the soul. Sin affected our ability to reason, make right decisions and keep emotions in proper balance. Our physical bodies have also been dramatically affected. In *The Word on Health,* Michael identified seven scriptural root causes to illness.

1. **Sickness unto Death.** Because we have mortal bodies and live in a fallen world, we will all die. Whether it is death by natural causes (i.e., old age or system failure) or due to a specific disease, we will all die from some cause. However, some religions believe that we are immortal. According to them, if we live "by the book," we will live forever, despite the fact that none of their teachers have ever succeeded in doing so. Others teach that we are god, or gods, and we just need to realize it (although none of their teachers have ever taken on the full attributes of God).

2. **Physical Causes.** These illnesses are not necessarily fatal; although, they come upon us for the same reason—that we are physical beings who live in a fallen physical world. Physical causes for disease range from acute, minor illnesses to those that are more chronic in nature. In many cases, these result from failure to live in harmony with natural law, such as when a person sustains an injury, eats a poor diet or gets inadequate exercise and rest.

3. **Chastisement**. These illnesses come upon us because of specific sin in our lives. For example, Paul warned the Corinthian church that many of its members had fallen sick or died because of the way in which they had dishonored the Lord at Communion. Paul was addressing Christians. In James 5:13-16, we are encouraged to call for the elders and ask for prayer if we are sick or suffering. Part of the healing process involves self-examination and confession of our faults (transgressions) to one another. These illnesses can lead to healing if the one who is suffering is willing to assume their own responsibility, pray and re-establish a righteous relationship with God.

4. **Wounded Spirit**. Solomon said, "The spirit of a man will sustain his infirmity; but a wounded spirit who can bear?" (Prov. 18:14, *KJV*)

Many people are physically sick with psychosomatic illnesses. These include some cases of depression, anxiety disorders, substance abuse, chronic fatigue, insomnia, Irritable Bowel Syndrome, ulcers, multiple chemical sensitivity/environmental illness and many others. We have seen many of these illnesses resolved when we help people repent and re-establish a righteous relationship with God. For others, their physical healing of psychosomatic illnesses is a matter of growth. They need to learn how to cast their anxiety onto Christ, overcome problems of depression by finding their hope in God or relieve stress by finding their peace in God. We are transformed by the renewing of our minds (Rom. 12:2) and that takes time. Some get sick because they have suffered from physical, mental, emotional and spiritual abuse. They need to overcome these abuses through forgiveness and faith in God. While there is no guarantee that we will not be victimized in our lifetime, we still have a choice. A choice to either (1) remain a victim or (2) overcome these adversities by establishing our freedom in Christ.

5. **Spiritual Maturity.** Sometimes a person has done nothing wrong and gets sick anyway. This happened to Job who was afflicted with boils from head to toe, not because of sin, but because he was so righteous that God allowed his integrity to be challenged by Satan himself. As seen in the life of Paul, sometimes weakness is used by God to keep us humble and usable for His service (see 2 Cor. 12:7-10). It is interesting to note that both Job and Paul were physically impaired for spiritual reasons allowed by God for a greater good.

6. **Glorify God Through Healing.** On numerous occasions in Scripture, individuals were healed in order that God would be glorified. For example, Jesus healed the paralytic who was lowered by his friends through the roof so that critical onlookers would know that he had the power to forgive sins (see Mark 2:1-12). In the case of a young man born blind, the Jewish leaders asked Jesus, "Rabbi, who sinned, this man or his parents, that he was born blind?" (John 9:2, *NKJV*). The Jewish community believed that sin was the cause of illness, but in this case Jesus said, "Neither this man nor his parents sinned . . . but this happened so that the work of God might be displayed in his life" (v. 9:3, *NIV*).

7. **Failure to Meet God's Conditional Promises.** Paul reminded the
Ephesian church (made up mostly of Gentile believers) that long life
is one of the rewards of honoring one's parents (see Eph. 6:1-3). Paul
indicated that this benefit of keeping the fifth commandment was
not only intended for the Israelites, recipients of the Mosaic Law,
but also for New Testament Gentile believers. Other conditional
promises in Scripture are also linked with good health and long life;
therefore, it stands to reason that the creator designed us to function a certain way. When we choose to live another way, we will
experience negative consequences. This is true for everything that is
created or man-made. For example, the computers we are using to
write this book will only work one way. If we study the manufacturer's handbook and learn its capacity, we would be able to generate
some incredible work. On the other hand, if we attempt to use the
computers in any other way than how the manufacturer has
designed them, they will not work. So it is with our physical and
mental health. Our potential in Christ is limited by how well we read
and understand the manufacturer's handbook—the Bible.[1]

RALPH AND AMY'S APPLICATION #2

The second step in evaluating a medical approach is to identify the religious
belief system, or worldview, upon which the approach was founded. This will
typically reflect the personal faith of its founder, which may be more difficult
to obtain. In our case study (presented in chapter 2), Amy's doctor was unable
to identify the religious affiliation of Reinhold Voll, the founder of the electrodermal approach that he was using. However, he pointed out that the technique
measured electrical energy along acupuncture meridians, and that it was a
Western version of traditional Chinese medicine (TCM), which is rooted in
Taoism.

George Goodheart, D.C., the founder of applied kinesiology (referred to by
some as muscle testing), is Roman Catholic. Nevertheless, he readily incorporated TCM meridian and acupuncture concepts into AK (see chapter 16).

As we will see in chapter 14, Taoism holds views that directly conflict
with biblical revelation. It disagrees with Christianity as to the nature of God,
creation, evil, the nature of man and, therefore, the cause and cure of illness.

Despite the fact that these distinctions have become somewhat obscured by Western terminology and high-tech computerized testing, they were, nevertheless, still a part of the medical practice of Amy's doctor. Looking through the grid of faith, Amy concluded that there were serious worldview problems with the approach she had begun to use.

MEDICINE'S FAMILY TREE

Wherever humans congregated throughout history, they developed religious beliefs to explain their existence, the cause of human suffering and how to recover their lost health and immortality. Each of these religions has therefore, in turn, given birth to medical paradigms to explain these ends.

The following diagram illustrates the genealogy of several major medical systems that will be addressed later in this book. For each system, the religious parentage from which that system was derived is identified. The chapters in which these approaches are addressed are indicated by parentheses. We recommend that you scan the chart now and then refer back to it as you read through the rest of the book.

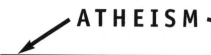

ATHEISM

Eastern Pantheism/monism

Taoism

Ayurveda (9)

TCM ~*200 B.C. (14)*
· acupuncture
· acupressure
· moxibustion
· macrobiotic diet
· Chinese herbs

Humoralism *(10)*
· *Pythagoras (530 B.C.)*
· *Hippocrates (420 B.C.)*
· *Galen (~A.D. 150)*

Allopathy *(10)*
(Until 1800s)

Iridology *(15)*
von Peczely (1864)

Reflexology *(15)*
Fitzgerald (1910)

Applied *(16)*
Kinesiology
George Goodheart (1964)

OCCULTISM — Psychic practices

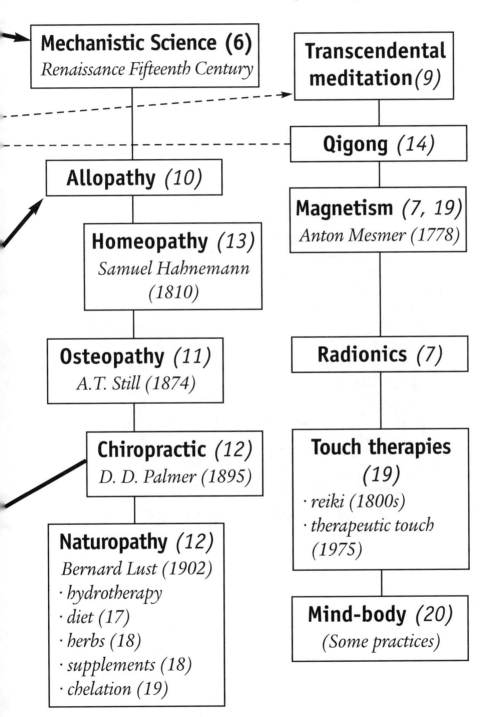

Mechanistic Science (6)
Renaissance Fifteenth Century

Transcendental meditation (9)

Qigong (14)

Allopathy (10)

Magnetism (7, 19)
Anton Mesmer (1778)

Homeopathy (13)
Samuel Hahnemann (1810)

Osteopathy (11)
A.T. Still (1874)

Radionics (7)

Chiropractic (12)
D. D. Palmer (1895)

Touch therapies (19)
· reiki (1800s)
· therapeutic touch (1975)

Naturopathy (12)
Bernard Lust (1902)
· hydrotherapy
· diet (17)
· herbs (18)
· supplements (18)
· chelation (19)

Mind-body (20)
(Some practices)

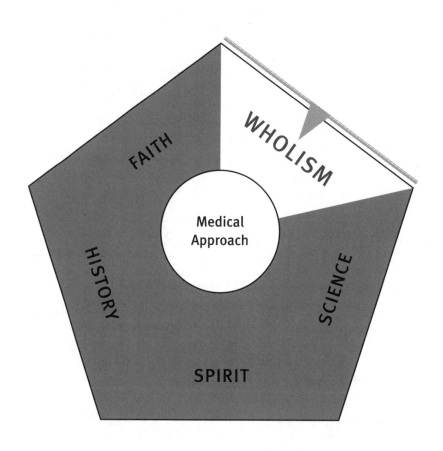

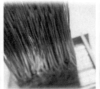

CHAPTER FIVE

EVALUATING THROUGH THE WHOLISTIC GRID

The head of a medical service in a great university hospital once said, "One should send for a minister as he sends for his doctor when he becomes ill." That is to say, God helps the sick in two ways, through the science of medicine and surgery and through the science of faith and prayer.

NORMAN VINCENT PEALE

There are some illnesses when the treatment of choice appears to be only physical. If you broke a leg, you probably wouldn't go see your pastor first. As a believer, you would probably pray and make your way to the emergency room at the local hospital. You might also call your pastor or Christian friends for prayer, and some might even volunteer to help you with household chores. But the basic need is to have the leg reset. On the other hand, there are illnesses that are clearly spiritual. If you are deeply weighed down by the gall of bitterness and the bondage of iniquity, you should go to God and then see your pastor if you don't know how to resolve the issues. If you seek help from the medical profession, they may prescribe medication that would temporarily mask the symptoms, but it wouldn't be a cure.

The problem is the twilight zone between the physical and the spiritual realms. In such cases, doctors may acknowledge your illness or pain, but they can't find any medical explanation for why you are suffering. Secular doctors may pass you off as a "head case" and recommend that you see a psychiatrist. Christian doctors face the same dilemma, but they feel uncomfortable recommending secular psychiatrists, who will likely medicate without therapy, or secular psychologists, who attempt therapy without any understanding of God, His ways and the spiritual world. Many of the illnesses in this twilight zone are psychosomatic or spiritual and require an integrated wholistic treatment plan.

There is also the need to integrate the psychological and the theological/spiritual. Trying to ascertain whether our problems are psychological or spiritual creates a false dichotomy. Our problems are usually always psychological. Our minds are always involved in the process of restoring good physical, mental, emotional and spiritual health. God always works through our minds and requires us to think maturely (see 1 Cor. 14:20), make rational choices (see Phil. 4:6-8) and study (see 2 Tim. 2:15). We are transformed by the renewing of our minds (see Rom. 12:2).

Along the same line of reasoning, our problems are also usually always spiritual. There is no time when God is not present. He "upholds all things by the word of His power" (Heb. 1:3). If God ceased to exist, so would we. We have to understand that the unseen spiritual world is just as real as the seen natural world, "for the things which are seen are temporal, but the things which are not seen are eternal" (2 Cor. 4:18). God is the ultimate reality. In addition, it is never safe to take off the armor of God. The possibility of being deceived, accused and tempted is a continuous reality. If we can accept that, then we will not polarize into psychotherapeutic ministries that ignore the reality of the spiritual world or conduct some kind of one-dimensional deliverance ministry that overlooks individual responsibility and the rest of reality. We have a whole God who deals with the whole person, and He will always take into account all reality.

There is also the tendency to see body illnesses as separate and isolated from our soul and spirit. For example, the physical symptoms of depression are not hard to assess. If your doctor is part of an HMO, and he has 10 minutes to talk to you and afterward he correctly diagnoses depression, what will he do? He or she will probably prescribe antidepressant medication. These doctors usually only have enough time to consider one dimension of your illness and quite possibly lack the training to consider anything other than physical causes and cures. But what is the cause of depression, and what is the cure? Some understand depression to be a biomedical or neurological problem, and the treatment of choice is antidepressant medication. Cognitive therapists understand depression to be caused by a negative view of ourselves, our circumstances and the future. In addition, most see depression as a reaction to losses in our lives and/or a learned sense of helplessness and hopelessness. If this is the case, can a secular psychologist or doctor provide sufficient answers? Can psychosomatic illnesses be resolved by manipulating brain chemistry only, or does a complete and sufficient answer need to take into account all the other dimensions of life?

As we work toward a complete answer, we need an integrated understanding of how the body, soul and spirit function together. Please refer to the following diagram for a complete overview.

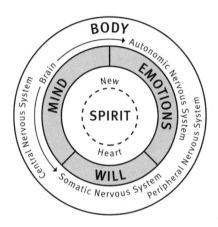

CENTRAL NERVOUS SYSTEM

In the original creation, God formed Adam and Eve from the dust of the earth and breathed into them the breath of life. This union of divine breath and earthly dust is what constituted Adam and Eve's physical and spiritual nature. Every human being is made up of an outer person and an inner person. In other words, we have a material self and an immaterial self. Our outer person, or material self, is what constitutes our physical body. Through our five senses we relate to the world around us. The inner person, or immaterial self, describes the soul/spirit of humanity. Created in God's image, we have the capacity to think, feel and choose.

As we were being fearfully and wonderfully made, it would only make sense that God would create the outer person to correlate with the inner person. The brain and mind correlation is obvious, but they are fundamentally different. Our brains are like organic computers that will return to dust when we physically die. However, if we are born-again believers, we will be mindfully present with the Lord. The mind is part of the soul, the inner immaterial person.

The brain is the capstone of the central nervous system, which also includes the spinal cord. Using the computer analogy, if the brain is the hardware, then the mind is the software. Neither the software nor the hardware can function without the other. The tendency in our Western world is to believe that if we are having some kind of mental or emotional problem, the cause is likely to be the hardware. Thus, medication would be the treatment of choice. We have been educated to first pursue every natural explanation for our illnesses and then seek every natural solution. If that doesn't work, then there is nothing left to do but pray or seek some alternative and unscientific treatment plan. Jesus instructed us to seek first His kingdom and His righteousness and all the rest will be added to us (see Matt. 6:33).

Scripture seems to indicate that mental and emotional issues are not primarily related to the hardware but rather to the software. Can we have hardware problems? Of course we can, and that needs to be considered if we are going to be wholistic. However, research is revealing that the precipitating cause is usually not neurological. A learned sense of helplessness and hopelessness can actually result in neurological changes (see Neil's book on depression entitled *Finding Hope Again,* Regal Books, 1999). Even secular researchers are acknowledging this concept. Martin Seligman, a noted researcher, reflected on the causes of depression:

> I have spent the last twenty years trying to learn what causes depression. Here is what I think. Bipolar depression (manic-depression) is an illness of the body, biological in origin and containable by drugs. Some unipolar depressions, too, are partly biological, particularly the fiercest ones. Some unipolar depression is inherited. If one of two identical twins is depressed, the other is somewhat more likely to be depressed than if they'd been fraternal twins. This kind of unipolar depression can often be contained with drugs, although not nearly as successfully as bipolar depression can be, and its symptoms can often be relieved by Electroconvulsive therapy.

But inherited unipolar depressions are in the minority. This raises the question of where the great number of depressions making up the epidemic in this country come from. I ask myself if human beings have undergone physical changes over the century that have made them more vulnerable to depression. Probably not. It is very doubtful that our brain chemistry or our genes have changed radically over the last two generations. So a tenfold increase in depression is not likely to be explained on biological grounds.

I suspect that the epidemic depression so familiar to all of us is best viewed as psychological. My guess is that most depression starts with problems in living and with specific ways of thinking about these problems.[1]

Peripheral Nervous System

Branching off from the central nervous system is the peripheral nervous system, which has two distinct channels.

Somatic Nervous System

One channel is the somatic nervous system, which regulates all of our muscular and skeletal movements. It is all the parts of our anatomy that we have volitional control over, meaning that if we have adequate physical health, we can mentally choose to move our limbs, smile and speak. Thus, the somatic nervous system correlates with our will. In other words, we don't do anything without first thinking it. The thought-action response is so rapid that one is hardly aware of the sequence. However, involuntary muscular movements occur when the system breaks down, as in the case of Parkinson's disease.

Autonomic Nervous System

The autonomic nervous system regulates all of our glands and correlates with our emotions. We don't have direct volitional control over the functioning of our glands. In the same way, we don't have direct volitional control of our emotions. We cannot will ourselves to like those who have disgusting character traits and behave poorly. However, we can choose to do the loving thing on their behalf, even though we don't like them, and this is what the Lord has commanded us to do. We cannot simply tell ourselves to stop feeling angry, anxious or depressed, because we cannot directly manage our emotions that way. But when we acknowledge that we are angry, anxious or depressed, we do have control over how we are going to express it. We can manage our behavior within limits, because that is something we have volitional control over. We have control of what we will think and believe, and that is what controls what we do and how we feel.

This reasoning follows when it becomes necessary to address angry, anxious or depressed people. Telling them that they shouldn't feel that way will only produce guilt, defensiveness (rationalization) and even retaliation. But we can encourage them to consider what it is they are believing and thinking; thereby, helping them learn to manage their behavior. For instance, we could say, "I know you are angry right now, but you don't have to take it out on others or yourself. Why don't you walk away and come back when you have cooled down and we can discuss it later." You will have as much success telling them to stop feeling angry as they will have trying to keep their autonomic nervous system from functioning.

Cognitive therapy is based on this understanding. People are doing what they are doing and feeling the way they feel because of what they have chosen to believe or think. Therefore, the primary focus should not be on trying to change behavior or feelings; it should be on trying to change beliefs and thoughts. "For as he thinks within himself, so he is" (Prov. 23:7). This is essentially repentance, which literally means a change of mind. Cognitive therapy from a secular perspective is insufficient for four reasons.

1. Changing what we believe from one pagan worldview to another means that we are still believing the lies of this world. It lacks the revelational truth that will set us free.
2. Even if we believe the words of Christ, without the life of Christ we lack the power to change. Remember, the Spirit gives life to the body (see Rom. 8:11).
3. Without understanding the potential spiritual battle that could be going on for our minds, cognitive therapy will not be wholistic or effective (see 1 Tim. 4:1; 2 Cor. 11:3).
4. The Lord Himself is the wonderful counselor. We simply lack any ability to bind up the brokenhearted and set the captive free. Apart from Christ we can do nothing (see John 15:5).

Anytime a counselor or doctor seeks to minister to another person, they are not the only two people present. God is always there, and there is a role that only He can play for patients and clients.

It is important to realize that what is causing the autonomic nervous system to respond is not the brain, and neither is the brain causing us to feel angry, anxious or depressed. It is the mind and the way it has been programmed. Neither do the circumstances of life or other people make us angry, but it is our perception of those people and events and how we interpret them that do, which is a function of our minds and how they have been programmed.

THE BRAIN-MIND CONNECTION

Let's apply the reasoning of the programmed mind to the problem of stress. When the pressures of life begin to mount, our bodies try to adapt. Our adrenal glands excrete hormones into our bloodstream enabling us to rise to the challenge. But if the pressure persists too long, stress becomes distress, our system breaks down and we become sick. Why do some people respond positively to stress while others get sick? Is it because one has superior adrenal glands? Some people are physically able to handle more pressure than others, but that is not the primary difference. The primary difference lies in the mind, not the body.

> Anytime a counselor or doctor seeks to minister to another person, they are not the only two people present. God is always there, and there is a role that only He can play for patients and clients.

Suppose two business partners are confronted with what one believes is a financial crisis. They have just lost a contract that they thought would bring them to a new level of prosperity. One partner wasn't a Christian, and he believed that this new contract would make him successful. Many of his personal goals would have been realized, but now his dreams are dashed. He responds in anger to all who try to console him and calls his lawyer to see if he can sue the company who broke the contract. His volatile reaction leads to many interpersonal conflicts, and he becomes a stress case and a stress carrier.

Unless this man learns to manage his thought life and change his beliefs to be more consistent with the Word of God, he will just become another statistic—perhaps one of the 500,000 Americans who suffer each year from a heart attack.[2] One such person was the famous psychologist John Hunter.

> He knew what anger could do to his heart: "The first scoundrel that gets me angry will kill me." Some time later at a medical meeting, a speaker made assertions that incensed Hunter. As he stood up and bitterly attacked the speaker, his anger caused such a contraction of blood vessels in his heart that he fell dead.[3]

The other partner in the above illustration is a Christian who deeply believes that success is becoming the person God created him to be. He believes that God will supply all his needs. Therefore, this loss has very little impact on him. He doesn't get angry and sees this temporary setback at work as an opportunity to trust in God. He believes that nobody or nothing on planet Earth can keep him from becoming the person God created him to be. That is God's goal for his life (see 1 Thess. 4:3).

One of these two partners is stressed out and angry while the other partner is experiencing very little stress and anger. Can faith in God have that kind of an effect on us? It can and it should. The primary difference between the two men is their belief system, not their physical capacity.

Physical Symptoms

Let's consider what is physically happening to the first partner as he reacts to the circumstances. The thoughts and feelings in his left cerebral cortex have already sent a signal deeper in the brain to hypothalamic nerve cells. The activated hypothalamic emergency system has stimulated sympathetic nerves to constrict the arteries carrying blood to his skin, kidneys and intestines. At the same time, the brain has sent a signal to the adrenal glands, and they are pumping large doses of adrenaline and cortisol into his bloodstream. As he fumes about the loss of a contract, his muscles tighten, his heart beats faster, and his blood pressure rises. In such a state, his blood would clot more rapidly in case of injury. Muscles at the outlet of his stomach are squeezing down so tightly that nothing can leave his digestive tract, causing it to become spastic, resulting in abdominal pains. The blood is directed away from the skin making it feel cool and clammy, and directed toward the muscles to facilitate a fight or flight response. He takes an antacid for his stomach and an aspirin to relieve his headache.

As the angry thoughts continue, his increased heart rate has pumped far more blood than is needed to just sit in his office. His body is prepared to spring into action, but there is no proper way to discharge his wrath. He is tempted to take it out on the rest of his employees, or yell at someone, and sometimes he does. The increased adrenaline stimulates his fat cells to empty their contents into the bloodstream. This provides additional energy that would be necessary if the situation required immediate action. But he is not active. He just sits there—fuming in his office—while his liver converts the fat into cholesterol. He has no one to fight and no where to take flight.

On the way home, he stops at the local watering hole for happy hour. After a couple hours of drowning his sorrows, he heads for home. His blood alcohol level makes driving dangerous, and it doesn't contribute to his health. If he continues to respond this way over time, the cholesterol formed from the unused fat in the bloodstream will accumulate. It then turns into plaque in the arteries that begins to block the blood flow. He is now a candidate for a heart attack. Imagine trying to help this person from only a physiological perspective!

> How our minds have been programmed is revealed by our belief system and subsequent behavior. It reflects our values and attitudes about life.

THE MIND REPROGRAMMED

Situations in life do not determine our physiological responses, nor is the secretion of adrenaline initiated by our adrenal glands. Instead, external events are picked up by our five senses and sent as a signal to our brains. The mind then interprets the data and chooses a path that determines the signal that is sent from the central nervous system to the peripheral nervous system. The brain cannot function any other way than how it has been programmed. That is why we are transformed by the renewing of our minds (see Rom. 12:2).

How our minds have been programmed is revealed by our belief system and subsequent behavior. It reflects our values and attitudes about life. Let's take another look at the angry man. He held certain beliefs about himself, life and life's values. Chances are his identity and sense of worth were tied into his career. He would consider himself a successful person if his business prospered and a failure if it didn't. He also believed that as an entrepreneur, he had to live the "high" life and experience the social esteem that comes from living in the right neighborhood and belonging to the right country club. Eventually this man's beliefs will destroy him and negatively affect those around him, including his family.

Dr. Edmund Bourne is a credible practitioner seeking to help those struggling with anxiety disorders. Dr. Bourne entered this field of study because he himself struggled with anxiety disorders. Five years after publishing *The Anxiety and Phobia Workbook*,[4] his own anxiety disorder took a turn for the worse. This caused him to reevaluate his own life as well as his approach to treatment. In 1998 he published a new book, which had this to say:

> The guiding metaphor for this book is "healing" as an approach to overcoming anxiety, in contrast to "applied technology." I feel it's important to introduce this perspective into the field of anxiety treatment since the vast majority of self-help books available (including my first book) utilize the applied technology approach. These books present—in a variety of ways—the mainstream cognitive behavioral methodology for treating anxiety disorders. Cognitive behavioral therapy reflects the dominant zeitgeist of Western society—a worldview that has primary faith in scientifically validated technologies that give humans knowledge and power to overcome obstacles to successful adaptation. . . . I don't want to diminish the importance of cognitive behavioral therapy (CBT) and the applied technology approach. Such an approach produces effective results in many cases, and I use it in my professional practice every day. In the past few years, though, I feel that the cognitive behavior strategy has reached its limits. CBT and medication can produce results quickly and are very compatible with the brief therapy, managed-care environment in the mental health profession at present. When follow-up is done over one- to three-year intervals, however, some of the gains are lost. Relapses occur rather often, and people seem to get themselves back into the same difficulties that precipitated the original anxiety disorder.[5]

His words read like a modern-day commentary of Colossians 2:8:

> See to it that no one takes you captive through philosophy and empty deception, according to the tradition of men, according to the elementary principles of the world, rather than according to Christ.

Dr. Bourne believes that "anxiety arises from a state of disconnection."[6] We agree, and the primary disconnection is from God, followed closely with being disconnected from the Body of Christ and other meaningful relationships.

We don't know whether Dr. Bourne has a saving knowledge of our Lord Jesus Christ, but in his own search for answers he came to the following conclusion:

> In my own experience, spirituality has been important, and I believe it will come to play an increasingly important role in the psychology of the future. Holistic medicine, with its interest in meditation, prayer, and the role of spiritual healing in recovery from serious illness, has become a mainstream movement in the nineties. I believe there will be a "holistic psychology" in the not too distant future, like holistic medicine, which integrates scientifically based treatment approaches with alternative, more spiritually based modalities.[7]

A BALANCED WORLDVIEW

We agree that there has been a movement toward wholistic health, but as mentioned earlier in the book, the spiritual base is not necessarily Christian. In fact, the prevailing

> We cannot expect our pastors to have the knowledge of medical doctors, nor can we expect our medical doctors to have the knowledge of our pastors.

religion in mainstream America is New Age. However, wholistic health requires the integration of our Christians beliefs in many disciplines. We cannot expect our pastors to have the knowledge of medical doctors, nor can we expect our medical doctors to have the knowledge of our pastors. And both will lack the counseling skills of a well-trained Christian therapist. Christ is the wonderful counselor, the great physician, and the author and finisher of our faith. He is the only perfectly balanced person to ever live on planet Earth, and we need to learn from Him and be led by Him. He occupies the center of the following diagram.

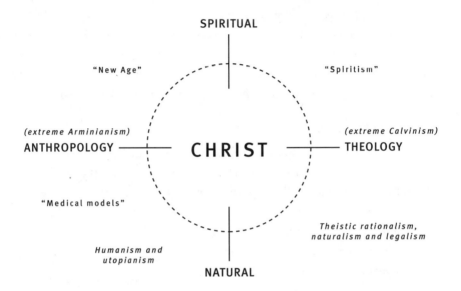

THE NATURAL EXAMINED

In working toward a biblical worldview and an integrated understanding of health and medicine, it is helpful to consider the balance between the natural and the spiritual. In addition, we need to understand the balance between the true nature of humanity (anthropology/psychology) and the true nature of God (theology) as well as their respective roles and responsibilities. The diagram does not pit one extreme against the other. The purpose is to show what happens when one dimension, or personality, is emphasized at the expense of the other.

Christ, the God-Man, is the true center. During His time on Earth, He had both the nature of God and the nature of humanity (see Phil. 2:5-8). He clearly acknowledged the reality of the spiritual world as well as the natural world. He is the only One who is perfectly balanced. The problem is we all think we are in balance. If we had enough self-awareness to know that we are seriously out of balance, we would be making serious moves to correct it. We cannot help but interpret the world from the viewpoint of our own education and experience. Wisdom, however, is seeing life from God's perspective. The circle around Christ represents the tolerance of belief within Christian orthodoxy. Anything outside the circle is not true or moral and needs to be confessed and renounced.

Medical Models and Humanism

The Western worldview has been skewed considerably toward the natural as compared with the rest of the world. Humanism has been the dominant worldview shaping the development of medicine and psychology. Secular schools perceive humankind as natural beings who live in a materialistic world. In keeping with this worldview, all public mental-health services maintain a strict separation between church and state. Consequently, the education and practices of medicine and counseling are located primarily in this lower left quadrant of the diagram. Most of our doctors and counselors, including Christians, have learned their medicine and psychology from the perspective of this quadrant. Liberal and neoorthodox churches also attempt to minister from this quadrant since they no longer rely on Scripture and a righteous relationship with God.

The shift of our Western culture is upward, but the spiritual nature of this shift is not predominantly Christian. It is New Age, and their practitioners have no sense of biblical revelation. We cannot overstate how profoundly their impact is being felt in education, business, medicine and psychology.

Theistic Rationalism, Naturalism and Legalism

Many of our churches are located in this lower right quadrant. Western rationalism and naturalism have seriously influenced our theology. Scholarship has been emphasized over godliness and spiritual formation in many of our seminaries. This can potentially reduce our walk with God to nothing more than an intellectual exercise. We can intellectually know all about God but not know Him personally. Legalism and dead orthodoxy have plagued the Church. We have captured the letter of the law but not the spirit of the law.

However, all this is changing—fundamentalism is dying in America. The fundamentals of our faith, however, haven't changed. They never will. Old traditions and customs that were formed from our culture more than from the Bible are being thrown off. Christians are less committed to institutions and even denominations, but they are often more committed to Christ and His kingdom. The Church is also shifting upward. Like any other movement, it is part good news and part bad news. The good news is people are discovering their spiritual identity in Christ and learning to live by faith in the power of the Holy Spirit. They are also discovering the reality of the spiritual world.

The bad news is that some people have moved into a subjective form of spirituality that has no objective base in Scripture. The Word has been replaced by the spirit, but which spirit? Without discernment, we can easily be deceived into thinking we are being led by the Holy Spirit, when in reality we are paying attention to a deceiving spirit (see 1 Tim. 4:1). Others have become demon chasers and spiritualize almost everything. Naturalism has been replaced by spiritism.

In this mixture of movement lies the ongoing debate between the Calvinists and the Arminians. Does our victory in Christ depend fully upon God (extreme Calvinism), or does it depend fully upon mankind (extreme Arminianism)? The Bible teaches that God is sovereign, but it also teaches that we have to fulfill our responsibilities. By faith we can trust God to be all that He says He is, and He will faithfully do all that He said He would do. The missing ingredient lies in our response to Him through repentance and faith. Therefore, if we repent and choose to live by faith according to what He says is true in the power of the Holy Spirit, we will live much healthier and longer.

RALPH AND AMY'S APPLICATION #3

We asked Amy's doctor if electrodiagnosis was part of a wholistic approach. Was it used to assess the whole person: spirit, soul and body? He answered by saying that information about the spiritual health, or psyche, of a person could be gleaned by this method—but only indirectly. He also confirmed our impression that electrodermal testing (also known as electroacupuncture) is a Western adaptation of traditional Chinese medicine. As we will see in chapter 14, TCM is a wholistic approach; however, its premises are inconsistent with Scripture. On the other hand, electrodermal diagnosis, a Western invention (or application)—as are many other aspects of Western medicine—is primarily biomedical. In other words, it focuses almost exclusively on the physical, not the spiritual.

And the very God of peace sanctify you wholly;
and I pray God your whole spirit and soul and body be
preserved blameless unto the coming of
our Lord Jesus Christ.

1 THESSALONIANS 5:23, *KJV*

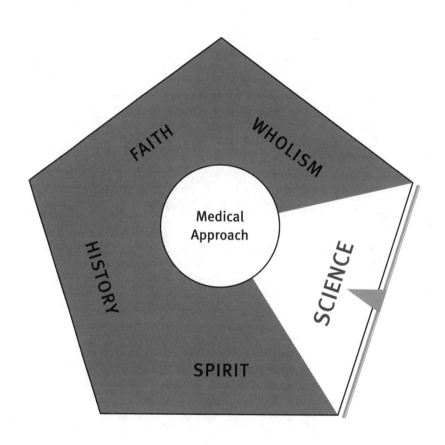

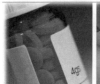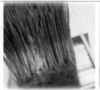

CHAPTER SIX

EVALUATING THROUGH THE GRID OF SCIENCE

I find it as difficult to understand a scientist who does not acknowledge the presence of a superior rationality behind the existence of the universe as it is to comprehend a theologian who would deny the advances of science. And there is certainly no scientific reason why God cannot retain the same position in our modern world that he held before we began probing his creation with telescope, cyclotron and space vehicles.

WERHNER VON BRAUN, PIONEER ROCKET SCIENTIST QUOTED IN THE PREFACE OF
CREATION: NATURE'S DESIGN AND DESIGNER

The fourth pillar upon which a biblical paradigm rests is natural law. The Judeo-Christian worldview is perhaps the only religious system that is completely compatible with science. Divine revelation and scientific research are not on a collision course. God created all things physical and endowed humankind with the capacity to study science for the purpose of discovering the wonders of the universe. God also commands man to be good stewards (see 1 Cor. 4:1-2). Those who think science is the final authority should read 50-year-old science books written by people who thought they were right at the time. The definition of science supports this hypothesis: The systematic observation of natural phenomena for the purpose of discovering laws governing those phenomena.[1]

Science is the study of nature with the intention of understanding, explaining and using natural law for the benefits of all. The laws of nature are physical laws that govern the physical universe. For example:

1. The circuits of the stars and planets are ruled by such precise law that the exact timing of sunrise and sunset can be determined years in advance and for centuries in retrospect.
2. The periodic table of elements lists all the basic building blocks of the universe as we know them. If we combine certain elements, such as hydrogen and oxygen, under certain atmospheric pressures and temperatures, we can predict with great accuracy what will happen. Below 32 degrees Fahrenheit at sea level, the combination of two parts hydrogen and one part oxygen will freeze and become ice.

THE LAWS OF NATURE

Laws that govern nature are consistent with divine revelation, because God's Word and His creation have the same author. Science looks for order and design, which are attributes of our creator—the God of order, not the author of confusion (see 1 Cor. 14:33,40). And He is the same yesterday, today and tomorrow (see Heb. 13:8). The Bible teaches that an omnipotent and omniscient creator spoke this universe into existence and then caused it to function according to the natural laws of science in a way that is always consistent with His Word.

I have made the earth, and created man upon it: I, even my hands, have stretched out the heavens, and all their host have I commanded (Isa. 45:12, *KJV*).

Bless the LORD, O my soul. O LORD my God, Thou art very great; Thou art clothed with honour and majesty. Who laid the foundations of the earth, that it should not be removed for ever. He appointed the moon for seasons: the sun knoweth his going down. O LORD, how manifold are thy works! in wisdom hast thou made them all: the earth is full of thy riches (Ps. 104:1,5,19,24, *KJV*).

It is tragic that the majority of scientists who reject Christianity have embraced the unproven theory of evolution, which denies the existence of the creator. Natural law presupposes a lawgiver. It is impossible to go from a state of chaos and disorder to fixed, universal law without a master designer. It is logically inconsistent to say you believe in natural law and not believe in God. Natural law cannot be separated from its creator.

Rule the Body

Natural law governs not only stars and planets; it also rules human health and physiology. For example, the development of the human being within the womb follows a specific, ordered process. Deviating from this pattern even minutely yields devastating results. The law of cellular respiration explains that our cells must burn oxygen and glucose for fuel; they will not survive with any other substance. Laws govern the production, regulation and action of hormones, as well as every other bodily process.

Rule the Universe

In addition, the laws of nature are universal. They apply to everyone regardless of who they are, where they live or whether or not they believe in them. If you stepped off the top of a building, you can predict the direction and speed you would fall because of the law of gravity. It wouldn't make any difference if you weren't aware of the law of gravity or you simply didn't believe in it. You'd still fall. You might think on the way down, *So far, so good,* but no amount of faith or willpower would reverse the inevitable consequence.

That is how some people live in regard to their physical health. Despite an exponential increase in the knowledge of our need for a wholesome lifestyle, we continue to violate what has been proven to be true. Such people are often shocked and bitterly disappointed later in life when they develop a disease that is a direct consequence of repeated transgressions of natural law. Apparently, they expected God to miraculously intervene and spare them the consequences of the laws He established. By the same irrational process, some will submit to bizarre treatment plans that simply are not consistent with God-given scientific principles.

Thus, a biblical medical paradigm not only acknowledges the laws of nature; it recognizes the need to live in harmony with them. How does one discover the natural laws that govern the universe? The answer is alluded to in the second half of the definition of "science." It concludes with, "the body of knowledge accumulated by such means."[2] "Such means" refers to the scientific method of investigation, which involves five specific steps.

1. State the problem;
2. Form a hypothesis;
3. Observe and experiment;
4. Interpret the data; and
5. Draw conclusions.

THE SCIENTIFIC METHOD

History attributes the birth of the scientific method of investigation to an English monk named Roger Bacon. Because there were so many errors in thinking at the time (even in the 1400s when Greek thought dominated Western Europe), Bacon saw the need to verify one's presumptions through research and experimentation. He also believed that understanding could be obtained without depending upon the ideas of those who were considered authorities in their respective fields. This form of logic became known as inductive reasoning, because it supposedly begins with simple observation with no allegiance to preconceived ideas. This was in contrast to knowledge being deduced from a known principle, as with Aristotle's deductive logic. Bacon's views were considered rebellious toward the establishment, and he was imprisoned for them.

Actually, the scientific method of investigation is much older than Bacon; it was first employed by Eve in the Garden of Eden (see Gen. 3).

1. **State the problem.** Eve was told not to eat of the tree of knowledge of good and evil. But the fruit looked tasty and appealing, and she wanted to be wise.
2. **Form a hypothesis.** Based upon the information given to her by the serpent, Eve hypothesized that she could partake of the fruit, become wise and have no adverse effect (i.e., she would not die).
3. **Observe and experiment.** She then conducted the experiment. She ate of the forbidden fruit and then repeated the experiment by giving it to her husband. Both experiments yielded the same results, showing the reproducibility of her findings.
4. **Interpret the data.** She noted that she was still standing, breathing, thinking and talking. She also noted that her husband was alive and

well. Furthermore, there was evidence that her knowledge had increased, because now, for the first time, she noticed that she and her husband were naked.

5. **Draw conclusions.** Eve may have initially concluded that her hypothesis was correct. She also must have concluded that there was no fixed, universal law that required her obedience to God since what He had predicted had not come true. If Eve's hypothesis had been true, then God's Word could not be trusted, and she would have had to determine truth for herself.

But she was dead wrong. She was not wiser; she was deceived. Her understanding and ability to reason had become corrupt. Furthermore, she had died spiritually, but did not know it due to her limited power to reason. The consequence she suffered was immediate disconnection from fellowship with her creator. In addition, the irreversible process of physical aging and dying had begun in her body.

A closer look at the scientific method of investigation reveals several inherent weaknesses and why it can produce conflicting, confusing and sometimes wrong results.

> If there is one thing that scientific research does confirm, it is that the more we learn, the more we realize we still don't know. Only God has all the facts.

Scientists Operate Without All of the Facts

Eve may have thought she had all of the facts she needed in order to form her hypothesis, conduct her experiment and draw her conclusions, but she didn't. First of all, she knew neither who the serpent was nor his intentions. Second, she did not know what true wisdom and knowledge were. Finally, she did not know what death was. She had never seen it or experienced it.

Scientific experimentation is always conducted with a limited perspective, and we will never know if we have all the necessary facts. Yes, knowledge is gained through systematic observation, but how do the scientists know if they are properly designing their research and interpreting their data? If there is one thing that scientific research does confirm, it is that the more we learn, the more we realize we still don't know. Only God has all the facts, "In whom are hidden all the treasures of wisdom and knowledge" (Col. 2:3).

The Scientific Method Is Not Truly Inductive

Eve did not simply reject the authoritative principles of her creator and start from scratch. Instead, she replaced them with false presuppositions (from the serpent) and used them as the basis for her experiment. The scientific method claims to be inductive—not simply reasoning from known principles. But this is not true. It is virtually impossible for man to function this way. Man always operates with a set of preconceived ideas and interprets what he or she sees through his or her own grid of education and experience. Man can't even think beyond his or her own vocabulary. *World Book Encyclopedia* explains it this way:

> The human mind probably does not actually solve problems in a systematic fashion. But, after the problem is solved, the scientist can use the scientific method to explain the problem and its solution in an orderly way.[3]

The question is not whether or not science operates from known principles, but from where those preconceived ideas are derived. Throughout most of its history, science has had a reputation for operating from false presuppositions. That is why science has repeatedly found the need to correct its faulty hypotheses and wrong conclusions.

Science Can Only Function Within the Physical Realm

Science can only measure what occurs in the physical realm (and that is limited by the scientists' instrumentation and their preconceived ideas of what measurements to consider). Since the natural world and the spiritual world interface and influence each other, science by itself cannot incorporate the whole picture. Natural law works for pure chemistry, but it doesn't work for the social sciences, since humanity has its own will. People can choose to cooperate or not. That is why human experimentation becomes a matter of probabilities, not absolutes. By definition, the scientific method of investigation ignores the reality of the spiritual world. God doesn't submit to our methods of investigation and, rest assured, Satan and his hoard are not going to cooperate either.

The Scientific Method of Investigation
Is Descriptive, Not Prescriptive

God had already warned Adam and Eve not to eat the fruit from the tree of knowledge of good and evil. He had already revealed that a law was in operation. However, they decided that they had to determine what was true for them. What a different world it would be if they had trusted God and never conducted the experiment. There are many people in science and medicine who practice blind faith in order to reveal to themselves what is true and what is not.

God has revealed Himself, His will and His ways through three means of revelation.

1. The psalmist wrote, "The heavens are telling of the glory of God; and their expanse is declaring the work of His hands" (Ps. 19:1). This is referred to as general revelation, which is discovered through empirical research and observation. Conclusions are based on reason and empirical studies.

2. The psalmist then mentioned special revelation. "The law of the LORD is perfect, restoring the soul; the testimony of the LORD is sure, making wise the simple" (Ps. 19:7). God's Word is special revelation. General revelation and special revelation are equivalent in what they reveal. General revelation is descriptive, but it does not answer the philosophical questions of why we are here. Research is helpful when it is descriptive—it helps us to identify what is—but it was never intended to be prescriptive. For example, measuring human depravity and then concluding that life was supposed to be lived that way is tragic. Special revelation defines and explains general revelation. It enables us to see life from God's perspective, and that is what wisdom is, as opposed to knowledge. Thus, we should always look at our observations through the grid of Scripture.

3. The ultimate revelation is Jesus, who said, "If you had known Me, you would have known My Father also; from now on you know Him, and have seen Him" (John 14:7).

Despite these limitations, science is a valid discipline and serves as the means to discover natural law. We see evidence of this in the life of King Solomon.

Considered one of the wisest men who ever lived, Solomon was known for his study of nature. He was a scientist.

> And Solomon's wisdom excelled the wisdom of all the children of the east country, and all the wisdom of Egypt. For he was wiser than all men . . . and his fame was in all nations round about. And he spake three thousand proverbs: and his songs were a thousand and five. And he spake of trees, from the cedar tree that is in Lebanon even unto the hyssop that springeth out of the wall: he spake also of beasts, and of fowl, and of creeping things, and of fishes. And there came of all people to hear the wisdom of Solomon, from all kings of the earth, which had heard of his wisdom (1 Kings 4:30-34, *KJV*).

Understanding creation gives greater insight into the creator and His ways. Perhaps that is one of the reasons for Solomon's wisdom. Science is not to be feared but embraced. God commanded man to subdue the earth and take dominion over it (see Gen. 1:28). Learning about creation is an important part of fulfilling that mandate. Science has tremendous value when it is conducted properly and when it subjects itself to biblical revelation.

> **Science has tremendous value when it is conducted properly and when it subjects itself to biblical revelation.**

We see the value of this in the life of Christopher Columbus. Despite the fact that conventional scientific opinion held that Earth was flat, Christopher Columbus decided he could sail around the world. Why? Because he placed his faith in Isaiah's revelation that God "sitteth upon the circle of the earth" (Isa. 40:22, *KJV*).[4]

Biblical revelation and what is observed in nature are compatible with one another when understood from God's perspective. If they appear to conflict with one another, there is a reason. For example, a recent study concluded that spanking was harmful to children. This directly conflicts with the "spare the rod and spoil the child" teaching (see Prov. 13:24; 19:18; 22:15). In such a case, one of two possibilities can be assumed.

1. **The research is wrong.** Perhaps the study did not differentiate between spanking in anger from spanking in a spirit of love. Maybe it did not differentiate between abuse and correction. Perhaps it used wrong parameters for determining what constituted spanking and what was harmful.

2. **Our understanding of the Scriptures is wrong or the Church has taken a wrong position not based in God's Word.** In our example, using the "rod of correction" (Prov. 22:15, *KJV*) does not mean that we have the license to abuse children. Instead, it probably means that using an instrument of discipline apart from the hand is appropriate in correcting aberrant behavior. Another example is how many centuries the Catholic Church agreed with Aristotle's conclusion that Earth was at the center of the universe. When Galileo's observations indicated otherwise, the Church had to re-examine its teaching. Nowhere does the Bible indicate that Earth is at the center of the universe. That was a faulty interpretation.

The same God who inspired the Judeo-Christian Scriptures also created the physical universe. As such, the Christian never needs to fear that the two will conflict with one another. Christians need to respect the sciences, and scientists need to embrace biblical revelation. If science is truly seeking to understand the laws of nature, then it must yield to the Lawgiver, the creator Himself. To fail to do so will only bring disastrous results similar to what Adam and Eve experienced.

HOW TO EVALUATE THE CREDIBILITY OF SCIENCE

While on a road trip several years ago, a friend noticed that his car seemed to develop a mind of its own. When he approached another vehicle and needed to pass, his car automatically accelerated. When he needed to exit the freeway to get gasoline, his vehicle seemed to know that it needed to slow down; it automatically decelerated on the exit ramp.

For several hours, all he had to do was steer the vehicle and apply the brakes. He was so excited about this "spirit-controlled car" that he couldn't wait to get back home and share what had happened with his family and friends. How embarrassed he was when I (Michael) revealed to him that it was not an invisible spirit, or force, that had been in control of his vehicle, it was me. When he refused to believe my claim, I took him outside and showed him how I had done it (I don't recommend this for winning friends).

During the trip, I had reclined my passenger front seat in order to rest. Upon doing so, I noticed a metal bar next to my toes that moved whenever the car changed speeds. Deciding to experiment (I don't recommend this for safety reasons either), I gently pulled back on the bar with my toes, confirming that I was able to make the car accelerate. All I had to do to slow the car down was to release pressure on the bar, the equivalent of removing foot pressure on the gas pedal.

Although my friend is an intelligent and rational person, his observations and conclusions were not accurate. Even though he was able to consistently reproduce his experience for several hours, his conclusions were wrong. Why? Because he did not realize that the information he had was inadequate to reach an accurate conclusion. When he was finally given all of the facts, he was able to correct his thinking and come to a proper conclusion.

So it is with scientific research. Some scientific observations are more accurate than others. In order to minimize error and help ensure that a proper understanding of nature is being achieved, scientists have attempted to establish rules for determining the quality of their research. We will summarize the rules by using a fictitious example of a clinical study researching the effectiveness of a new drug for high blood pressure.

1. **The size of the study.** In general, the more people studied, the more reliable the results. A study showing that a new drug effectively reduced blood pressure in 2,000 patients would be considered much more valid than one that only observed its effectiveness in six patients. This is a consistent error that is made more often among laypeople than scientists. If just one person is cured in a church, the whole church may try the same remedy.

2. **Placebo-controlled.** In any given study, it is expected that up to one-third of the patients will experience a reduction in their blood pressure simply because they believe that the drug is working. This is known as the placebo effect. In order to compensate for this, study participants are divided into two groups, with half receiving the real drug and half receiving a placebo (a copy of the real thing, but it doesn't have any inherent biochemical activity). Note: The placebo effect occurs frequently in psychosomatic illnesses. If taking the

medicine gives a person a sense of hope, it may have a positive effect even though the drug did nothing to affect the body chemistry.

3. **Randomization.** Since everyone in the study would naturally prefer to get the real medicine, the individual members are *randomly assigned* to either the experimental group (they receive the real drug) or the control group (they get the placebo). You cannot predict results for the general population unless there is a fair sampling.

4. **Blind studies.** When patients in a research study do not know if they are receiving the real drug or placebo, the study is said to be *single-blind*. Not only can patients be biased, scientists can be as well, especially those who would really like to see a particular result come from the study. Therefore, the best studies are those in which neither the doctor nor the patients know which treatment any particular subject is receiving. These studies are said to be *double-blind*.

5. **The design of the study.** The best studies will be those that are properly structured to control for certain factors that might influence the issue(s) being addressed. For example, high blood pressure tends to be more common in those who are smokers, heavy coffee drinkers, overweight, experiencing stress and older. If the experimental group has 90 percent of the smokers, coffee drinkers, overweight, stressed-out and elderly people, it would be quite easy for the drug to look effective when compared to the control group.

6. **Length of the study.** Generally speaking, the longer the study, the better the opportunity to get a more complete picture of a drug's effects and side effects. Unfortunately, longer studies are more difficult to complete and much more expensive. They also run the risk of many other factors being introduced into the study.

The double-blind, randomized, placebo-controlled study is the gold standard of the scientific medical profession. It is the most reliable way to determine which treatments are most effective. It is not infallible, and studies examining the same problem often come up with conflicting results. One of the major reasons for this is the fact that people are complex beings. It is very difficult to have exactly the same set of circumstances in different individuals. That is why researchers also have to control other factors that might influence the outcome of the study. Since new discoveries are being made every day as to the cause and nature of diseases, it is easy to see how complex these research studies can become and how difficult it is to authoritatively state one's conclusions.

Science is a wonderful profession, and its discoveries have provided us with countless benefits and conveniences. However, science and the scientific method must not usurp the place of God. Only God is to be worshiped, and scientific study should be conducted with a reverent respect for the creator.

RALPH AND AMY'S APPLICATION #4

When asked if there were scientific studies that document the effectiveness of electrodermal testing (see chapter 2), Amy's chiropractor replied that most of the research on it was being conducted in South Africa. He also mentioned a Florida medical doctor who had lost his license (apparently for using this approach) and was now devoting his career to researching this approach.

Next, I (Michael) went to the National Library of Medicine's website (www.nlm.nih.gov) to look for articles on the subject. There I clicked on "Health Information" and searched a variety of terms, including "electrodermal," "electrodiagnosis," "Voll," "EAV" and so on. Here is what I found.

1. There were only a small number of controlled trials examining the practitioner's approach. Of these, most dealt with psychology, such as the measurement of skin resistance in response to stress, lie detection, etc. This is based upon a different concept than acupuncture points and meridians.

2. I found only two studies that tested electrodermal testing as a diagnostic tool in nonpsychological disease. Both dealt with allergies, and both were out of the same hospital in England. The studies even involved some of the same researchers. A 1997 study found it to work well.[5] However, they must have had second thoughts, because a 2001 study looking at the same question concluded that the Vegatest was worthless in diagnosing allergies to dust mites or cat dander.[6]

3. And finally, I found no studies out of South Africa, which contradicted what the practitioner told Amy, Ralph and me.

Looking at electrodermal testing (i.e., electroacupuncture) through the grid of science, we concluded that this approach to diagnosing disease is questionable at best.

FINAL THOUGHTS

Just because an approach does not have good scientific evidence to support it does not mean that it should be automatically discarded. For one thing, the approach may be so new that there has not been adequate opportunity for studies to be conducted. Second, the scientific community has a historical reputation for strongly opposing major paradigm shifts in its thinking. For example, Doctors Lister and Semmelweiss were vehemently attacked for suggesting that poor medical hygiene promoted the spread of disease.

Finally, it may surprise you to learn that only a small percentage of procedures and practices in modern medicine have been clearly proven to be effective by good scientific research. Most of what we do as physicians is done because it is what we were taught to do and not necessarily done because it has been clearly proven beyond any reasonable doubt that it is the best solution. In his insightful article addressing why chelation therapy is not more widely accepted, Tulane University professor Dr. James Carter points out a report by the Office of Technology Assessment (a branch of Congress) which concluded that only 10 to 20 percent of the procedures currently used in medical practice have been shown effective by controlled trials. Of those 10 to 20 percent in which controlled trials had been conducted, the report also noted that much of the research was seriously flawed.[7]

While these numbers appear unbelievably low, Dr. Carter points out a perplexing double standard in which the medical establishment rejects many new or alternative ideas on the basis that the approaches are unproven (when in reality it is probably because they conflict with its own convention), while at the same time ignoring the fact that much of its own practice is unproven as well. This is one of the reasons why the grid of science is only one of five grids that is employed in evaluating a medical approach. The study of nature (science) is wonderful, but our knowledge is incomplete. What we do know tends to be distorted by personal bias and preconvention. In and of itself, science alone is an inadequate standard of measurement.

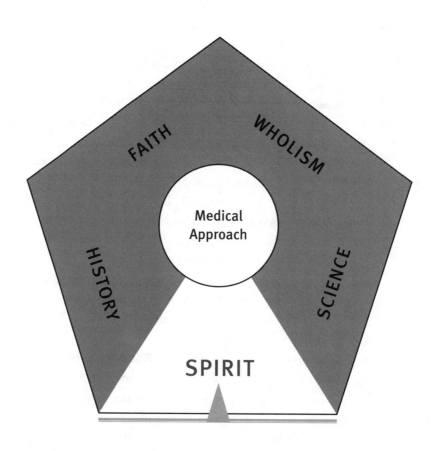

CHAPTER SEVEN

EVALUATING THROUGH THE GRID OF SPIRITUAL DISCERNMENT

Spiritual power is a force which history clearly teaches has been the greatest force in the development of man. Yet we have been merely playing with it and never really studied it as we have the physical forces.

CHARLES P. STEINMETZ, GERMAN-AMERICAN ELECTRICAL ENGINEER,

INTERVIEW WITH ROGER W. BABSON

Gucci, Rolex, Stradivarius—just the mention of these names and one thinks of quality. These brands represent the best in their fields, and their products are so expensive that only the wealthy can afford them. And since ownership communicates a message of prosperity, many people in the world desire to own these products. The problem is that the price is so high that most will not pay it. As a result, there exists a black market of brand-name look-alikes. While these illegal products look like the genuine article, they are not. Even so, they derive their value from the real thing by how closely their appearance mimics that of the brand-name product.

So it is in the spiritual realm, which is referred to by the apostle Paul as the "heavenly places" (Eph. 2:6; 3:10). The Scriptures teach us that there is but one God; all other would-be gods are imposters. The Bible also teaches us that we were designed by God to worship Him and to have a personal relationship with

Him. Since we are incomplete without Christ and were never designed to live independently of God, we have this spiritual vacuum inside, an inner longing to be complete. Only "in Christ" are we made complete (Col. 1:28; 2:10). Many

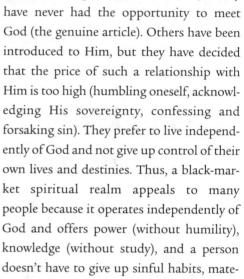

We are incomplete without Christ and were never designed to live independently of God; we have this spiritual vacuum inside, an inner longing to be complete.

have never had the opportunity to meet God (the genuine article). Others have been introduced to Him, but they have decided that the price of such a relationship with Him is too high (humbling oneself, acknowledging His sovereignty, confessing and forsaking sin). They prefer to live independently of God and not give up control of their own lives and destinies. Thus, a black-market spiritual realm appeals to many people because it operates independently of God and offers power (without humility), knowledge (without study), and a person doesn't have to give up sinful habits, materialism and autonomy. However, all it costs is our soul. And unfortunately, too many lost souls are being pulled into these spiritually dangerous faiths and belief systems.

THE REAL THING?

Eastern Substitutes

In ancient China, the realm of the spirit was identified as a "life force" that supposedly permeated the universe and all living beings. To this day, the Chinese culture still attempts to access and benefit from this force through a variety of means, including seasonal (macrobiotic) diets, herbs, breathing exercises, meditation and medical approaches designed to open "blocked" energy channels. The Hindus call this life energy "prana." Since they view prana as the highest form of consciousness or intelligence, great emphasis is placed upon altering one's own level of consciousness in order to contact the prana state through transcendental meditation (TM) and yoga.[1]

The Greeks initially equated this life force with the healing power of nature and later conceived of it as a breath, ether or spirit. Then these supernatural concepts were challenged during the Renaissance. A flood of scientific discovery led scientists to explain all of life on a purely natural basis. This "man is nothing more than chemicals that operate on the basis of physical law" model endured for a season, but soon its inadequacies also became apparent. In response, elite universities of the eighteenth century developed the concept of "vitalism," which is defined as "the proposition that more is needed to explain life than just physical or mechanical laws."[2]

Proponents of vitalism contend that there is some unseen property that is present during life and is removed from the body at the time of death (notice the similarity to the biblical concept of human spirit). Some philosophers and scientists felt that this invisible property was inherently physical; others believed it to be spiritual. Eventually, the invisible property became viewed as two sides of the same coin and referred to respectively as lower and higher mesmerism. The reason for this terminology is traceable to an unusual eighteenth-century physician Frank Anton Mesmer.

Mesmer's "Energy"

Mesmer was born in Austria in 1734, just 21 years before Samuel Hahnemann, the founder of homeopathy. Like Hahnemann, Mesmer studied medicine in Vienna. His ideas were probably derived from George Ernest Stahl (1660-1734), the founder of animism, who maintained that the source of all vital movement was the "anima," which governed the organism and disappeared at death. Mesmer embraced the idea of animism and hypothesized that magnetic therapy could correct erratic flow of this invisible energy.[3]

Initially, he used magnets to bring about this correction. But eventually he came to believe that his own magnetic power was able to exert the necessary effect upon his patients. He proposed that doctors function as mediums, meaning that their healing life force passed through them to their patients. This did not sit too well with Mesmer's colleagues, who angrily rejected him and his strange theory known as "animal magnetism." Looking for a more receptive atmosphere, Mesmer moved to Paris in 1778 where his healing events became a popular attraction. In a typical session, patients stood in a circle touching one another while going through a ritual in which the magnetic flow supposedly went through their bodies, causing some to faint, utter strange voices or even go into convulsions.

Mesmer created such a stir that a committee was eventually commissioned by the French government to investigate his claims. The nine members included

Antoine Lavoisier (the famous chemist), Dr. Frank Guillotine (whose name is associated with the execution device that was later applied to Lavoisier's neck) and the popular scientist and American ambassador Benjamin Franklin. This distinguished group designed several experiments to test the validity of magnetic therapy. For example, since patients claimed that they could feel the magnetism, they were blindfolded and then asked whether or not they were being exposed to it. The committee concluded that Mesmer's therapy was purely suggestive and that no genuine healing took place. It eventually fell out of favor, but his name and the concepts of vitalism and hypnotism persist in medicine today.[4]

SPIRITUAL OR PHYSICAL—OR JUST A CONTINUUM?

Some modern alternative medicine approaches show a strong similarity to that of Mesmer's approach. These are referred to as higher mesmerism. A contemporary American textbook openly acknowledges that these practices involve contact with the occult.

> The trance states of higher mesmeric traditions were used to contact **noncorporeal realities** [i.e., spiritual beings, emphasis added]. Healing dispensations, medical diagnosis, or medical advice were a common product of "tuning in," as was clairvoyance, spirit sightings, levitations . . . table turning, spirit tapping, and spirit photographs. . . . This spiritualist movement was later reincarnated in various theosophical and occult movements in today's New Age scene. . . . Past lives therapy are involved with a panoply of spiritual beings *detectable by mesmeric trances*, currently spoken of as altered states of consciousness, channeling, higher states of awareness, or transmission of spiritually evolved beings.[5]

In contrast, adherents to lower mesmerism explain that the life force is not describing something that has a spiritual nature but a physical nature. They deny contact with the occult. Instead, they use terms such as "vital force" or "electromagnetic energy." But the same textbook cited above contends that these are not two distinct entities, only a difference in terminology.

Lower mesmeric forms of healing energy are easily recognized in the contemporary alternative therapies that speak of an electromagnetic dimension which can become depleted or unbalanced . . . [causing] the blockage of energy flow, requiring physical or spiritual cleaning in order for healing to occur. Alternative therapies—such as therapeutic touch, laying on of hands, polarity, paranormal healing, and the countless individual psychic, auric, and psionic healers—while often unaware of their heritage, all bear the characteristic mesmeric style of manipulating unseen and refined forces that evade biomedical detection.[6]

Whether higher or lower mesmerism, qi (chee), prana or vital force, all bear one thing in common: They substitute their own hypotheses for what the Bible refers to as the spiritual realm.

The earliest reference to universal energy was in India, 5000 B.C. Since then, many cultures have developed rich philosophies and healing traditions around this concept. Some terms used to describe the phenomenon are *prana* in India; *qi* in China, Thailand and Japan; and *mana* in Hawaii. In 500 B.C., Pythagoras called it *vital energy*. Mesmer who developed hypnosis in the 1800s, named it *animal magnetism*. *Some believe it is the essence of the Christian holy spirit* (emphasis added).[7]

In other words, this statement implies that Christians' belief in the Holy Spirit is a case of mistaken identity. Just because someone denies the existence of God does not mean that He does not exist. Redefining terms or claiming that someone or something does not exist does not make it so. God's existence is independent of man's belief.

As Christians, we assert that God does exist, and that there is a vast spiritual realm of good and evil. The Bible gives us numerous examples of the devastation wreaked upon human lives from the influence of evil spirits. Satan, the "father of lies" (John 8:44), is described as a thief who "comes only to steal, and kill, and destroy" (John 10:10). Therefore, the apostle Peter warns us to "be of sober spirit, be on the alert. Your adversary, the devil, prowls about like a roaring lion, seeking someone to devour" (1 Pet. 5:8).

Therefore, our fifth and final step in a biblical test of medicine is to ascertain whether or not the spiritual realm is involved in the medical practice and the belief behind it. This requires spiritual discernment along with good biblical theology. In that regard, perhaps you can relate to my (Neil) personal journey in this critical area.

CAN YOU RELATE?

I was an aerospace engineer before I became a Christian. I thought science was the answer; I believed there was a natural explanation for everything and, therefore, a natural answer for the problems of humanity. Then I became a Christian and attended a good seminary. I learned about the kingdom of God, but I was taught very little about the kingdom of darkness. I learned how to explain almost every human problem on the basis of the fallen world and the struggle with the flesh, but not with the devil.

I have since gone through a lot of paradigm shifts in my thinking and understanding of reality and the Word of God. Scripture hasn't changed, but I have. I now believe that the essential battle from Genesis to Revelation is between the kingdom of God and the kingdom of darkness, between Christ and the Antichrist, between the Spirit of Truth and the father of lies, between true prophets and false prophets, and between good angels and evil spirits. I understand a little better what Paul meant when he wrote that, "our struggle is not against flesh and blood, but against the rulers, against the powers, against the world forces of this darkness, against the spiritual forces of wickedness in the heavenly places" (Eph. 6:12). Consequently, I believe that every Christian needs to put on the armor of God and "be on the alert with all perseverance and petition for *all* the saints" (Eph. 6:18, emphasis added). I believe we all need to "be of sober spirit, be on the alert. Your adversary, the devil, prowls around like a roaring lion, seeking someone to devour" (1 Pet. 5:8).

The Church is defined by the presence of the Holy Spirit who indwells every believer. He will lead us into all truth and enable us to be discerning in these latter days. This is critical, since Paul warned us about these times. "The Spirit clearly says that in later times some will abandon the faith and follow deceiving spirits and things taught by demons" (1 Tim. 4:1, *NIV*). Paul also describes who we formerly were, which still describes those who are outside the kingdom of God. "And you were dead [spiritually] in your trespasses and sins, in which you formerly walked according to the course of this world, according to the prince of the power of the air, of the spirit that is now working in the sons of disobedience" (Eph. 2:1-2). That spirit at work in the lives of unbelievers is what allows Satan to continue functioning as the god of this world and explains why "the whole world lies in the power of the evil one" (1 John 5:19).

Our heavenly Father is a spiritual being and not a higher power or cosmic force. We relate to Him personally. Fallen humanity tries to depersonalize God, because an impersonal god doesn't have to be served. With the same reasoning, orthodox Christianity has always acknowledged the reality of a personal devil as opposed to an evil force. You can resist a person but not an inanimate force. Therefore, pagans prefer to think of the spiritual world as a force, or energy, that has no moral basis for what is right or wrong.

Primitive animistic or spiritistic cultures try to manipulate the spiritual world through their shamans and witch doctors. They try to appease the deities by leaving offerings of fruits and vegetables. Some have offered human or animal sacrifices, which is a direct counterfeit of Christianity and the sacrifice that Christ made on our behalf. These false religious systems all require people to sacrifice to their gods, but our God sacrificed for us. They don't know that Jesus defeated the devil and disarmed him. If they came to Christ, they would have power and authority over the kingdom of darkness.

HOW CAN I EVALUATE THE FIFTH GRID— SPIRITUAL DISCERNMENT?

We move on then to the most important of our five grids and this question: If the practice impinges upon the spirit realm, is the spirit that is involved the Holy Spirit? In our five-part test, this question *must* be answered in the affirmative if the approach is to be considered. If a spirit is involved, and it is not God's Spirit, it is not to be believed (see 1 John 4:1) but rejected (see Jas. 4:7). How do we know if the spirit is of God? The answers to the following questions will help reveal the spirit behind the power that is at work:

1. What is the practice?
2. What does the spirit confess?
3. What is the fruit?

What Is the Practice and Does Scripture Forbid It?

For our own protection, God has forbidden contact and cooperation with Satan and his kingdom and has banned any activity that would lead to that end. We are instructed not to consult mediums and spiritists (see Lev. 19:31). If we did, God would turn His face against us and cut us off from the rest of His people (see Lev. 20:6). In the Promised Land, mediums and spiritists were to be put to death. In addition, Moses warned us about practicing any form of spiritism or occultic activity.

> There shall not be found among you anyone who makes his son or his daughter pass through the fire, one who uses divination, one who practices witchcraft, or one who interprets omens, or a sorcerer, or one who casts a spell, or a medium, or a spiritist, or one who calls up the dead. For whoever does these things is detestable to the LORD; and because of these detestable things the LORD your God will drive them out before you (Deut. 18:10-12).

Witches, mediums and spiritists—certainly no Christian would knowingly get involved with such people. However, many Christians do. Most believers are not consciously aware of the counterfeit activity in which they are involved. Just change the names from demon to spirit guide and medium to channeler, and a naive and undiscerning society seems to think it is okay. Many Christians are being deceived into believing that a practice is innocuous, when in fact it involves contact with the occult. As an example, let's consider how the practice of divination was addressed in the Bible.

> Through divination mediums attempt to discern future events *(or, with respect to medicine, we add "the cause and treatment of illness")*. They do so through trances and visions, or they will sometimes use physical objects. These attempts were varied: (1) *rhabdomancy*, the throwing of sticks or arrows into the air (Ezekiel 21:21; cf. Hosea 4:12); (2) *hepatoscopy*, examination of the liver or other organs of an animal (Ezekiel 21:21); (3) *teraphim*, images used for divination (1 Samuel 15:23; Ezekiel 21:21; Zechariah 10:2); (4) *necromancy*, communication with the dead (Deuteronomy 18:11; 1 Samuel 28:8; 2 Kings 21:6) which was condemned

in the law and the prophets (Leviticus 19:31; 20:6; Isaiah 8:19-20); (5) *astrology*, reading the stars and coming to conclusions on the basis of their positions and relations to each other (Isaiah 47:13; Jeremiah 10:2); (6) *hydromancy*, divination with water, done either by noting the reflections, or inducing a trance by this means. In order to confuse his brethren, Joseph had his servants suggest the goblet found in their sacks was for that purpose (Genesis 44:5,15); no approval of such a practice is implied. God sternly condemns all means of seeking hidden knowledge and knowledge of the future apart from His divine revelation.[8]

These occult practices have one thing in common: They attempt to gain knowledge or power from the supernatural realm apart from God. The kind of knowledge being referred to here is esoteric knowledge that does not come from diligent study or reason. It is knowledge that comes directly from some ungodly supernatural source. The lure of knowledge and power has enticed more than one victim. Knowledge is important because knowledge is power. Notice that all occultic practices deal either with the future or the mind but usually both. They want you to believe that they can know your mind or the future perfectly, but that is not true. Only God can do that.

Obviously, most believers know better than to get involved in paranormal or psychic experiences such as trances, visions, hypnosis, etc., in which control of the mind is surrendered to an unknown entity. But when the practitioners use physical objects, it tends to obscure the occult nature underlying the practice of divination. There are three salient characteristics of a practice that involves contact with the occult.

1. The purpose of the activity is to gain *information* or *power*.
2. The *immaterial* (i.e., the spirit, supernatural or energy realm) is asked to manifest itself (i.e., give an answer) through a *material* object.
3. The question is usually (but not always) framed so as to obtain a simple *yes* or *no* answer.

How Is Divination Practiced in Medicine?

In medicine, the occult nature of questionable practices can be further obscured by medical concepts and technology. But if you keep the three spirit questions in mind, you will see them form a recurring theme in the following actual-case scenarios.

A patient is asked by her physician to lie on her back on a treatment table. Her doctor stands at the foot of the table and grasps one of her ankles with each hand. He then asks her body to tell her what illness it has. "Do you have a disease of the kidneys?" If no movement is detected in her legs, the answer is no. Conversely, if one leg becomes longer or shorter than the other, the answer is yes.

A lock of hair is sent to an out-of-state healer who purportedly has the ability to test this substance and determine the patient's diagnosis. But instead of running the hair through an analyzer to evaluate its physical content (such as heavy metals), he hangs a pendulum over it, sequentially asking questions as to the patient's illness. "Is there heart trouble?" If the answer is no, the pendulum does not move. If the answer is yes, the pendulum swings.

There is no logical explanation for how a physical object, such as a leg or a lock of hair, can answer questions verbally presented to it. It should be obvious that in each of these cases, the supernatural/immaterial realm is being asked to provide information to the physical/material realm. Rhabdomancy uses sticks, pendulums or other objects as mediums for divining forms from the supernatural. But what difference does it make if what is being used to obtain information from the supernatural is a stick, a pendulum, a leg, a muscle or any other instrument? It's all potentially divination. And if it is divination, then it is an abomination to God.

What an insult it must be to God to see people throwing sticks in the air, slaughtering animals, checking leg lengths and dangling pendulums over locks of hair, all for the purpose of getting information He already knows. How much better to be born again into God's family through faith in Christ and to have Him put His Spirit within us to lead and guide us. All we have to do is ask for His guidance. And if He chooses to be silent, we are better off ignorant than to contact a counterfeit spirit whose very nature is to lie.

WHAT DOES THE SPIRIT CONFESS?

The primary test of orthodoxy is given in 1 John 4:1-3:

> Beloved, do not believe every spirit, but test the spirits to see whether
> they are from God; because many false prophets have gone out into the

world. By this you know the Spirit of God: every spirit that confesses that Jesus Christ has come in the flesh is from God; and every spirit that does not confess Jesus is not from God; and this is the spirit of the antichrist, of which you have heard that it is coming, and now it is already in the world.

The primary issue that John is addressing is the problem of gnosticism. The gnostics believed that everything in the physical realm was evil and everything in the spiritual realm was good. They denied that Jesus is God incarnate and that He came in the flesh, and so do the modern cults of the world. Lordship (acknowledging or yielding to the lordship of Jesus) is another test (see 1 Cor. 12:3). New Age practitioners and cult leaders will acknowledge a belief in Jesus, but they are preaching Him another way. Consequently, they receive a different spirit and a different gospel (see 2 Cor. 11:3-4). In some cases, the practitioner, or spirit, should be asked directly, "Do you confess Jesus Christ as the Son of God, who has come in the flesh? And do you now confess Him as the Lord of your life?" However, they can lie in their response. Many will say they believe in Jesus, but that does not automatically amount to an endorsement of the practice.

Suppose a missionary girl fell and sustained a gash in her leg. Her parents took her to the nearest village where there was a non-Christian native doctor. After examining her wound, he cleaned it and applied an herbal salve to enhance clotting. Once the bleeding stopped, he cleaned the wound again and applied a bandage to hold the edges together while it healed. Despite the fact that this practitioner was not a believer, from all appearances there was no spiritual danger. He was treating a physical injury with a physical remedy that was needed by the girl's body to stop the bleeding.

On the other hand, what if the doctor pulled out a bloodstone (which is used in occultism for bleeding problems) and began uttering strange verses from some unknown source while waving the object over the girl's cut? This presents an entirely different scenario. Now the practitioner is invoking the spiritual realm.

Let's consider a third possibility. What if the doctor professes to be a Christian, and yet, he employs the latter approach just described? Does the fact that he professes to be a Christian neutralize the occult influence that would be involved if the practitioner were not a believer? It is hard for some to believe that a Christian could actually be a channel for the enemy, but unfortunately, it is possible. Good people can be deceived and can spread their deception; that is why the Lord ordered them to be cut off from the rest of His people so that others would not be contaminated (see Lev. 20:6). We (Neil and Michael) have both seen deceived Christians bring New Age medical practices into the church or recommend them to other believers.

> Just because practitioners claim to be Christians does not guarantee that everything they do is compatible with biblical faith.

Just because practitioners claim to be Christians does not guarantee that everything they do is compatible with biblical faith. On the contrary, we often hear of a practice that is clearly pagan or even occult-like, only to learn that the individual who is espousing it is a believer. Peter did say, "there will also be false teachers among you, who will secretly introduce destructive heresies, even denying the Master who bought them" (2 Pet. 2:1). There are two ways to recognize false teachers.

1. They "despise authority" (2 Pet. 2:10). They have an independent spirit and won't answer to anyone.
2. Their immorality will eventually reveal who they are. "For such men are false apostles, deceitful workers, disguising themselves as apostles of Christ. And no wonder, for even Satan disguises himself as an angel of light. Therefore it is not surprising if his servants also disguise themselves as servants of righteousness; whose end will be according to their deeds" (2 Cor. 11:13-15).

WHAT IS THE FRUIT?

Does the practitioner and/or the patient exemplify the fruit of the Spirit or the works of the flesh? Paul said, "the fruit of the Spirit is love, joy, peace, patience, kindness, goodness, faithfulness, gentleness, self-control" (Gal. 5:22-23). Conversely, "the deeds of the flesh are . . . immorality, impurity, sensuality, idolatry, sorcery, enmities, strife, jealousy, outbursts of anger, disputes, dissensions, factions, envying, drunkenness, carousing" (Gal. 5:19-21). Be careful, however. Christians can still live according to the flesh by their own choice. New believers will exhibit many characteristics of the flesh, and so will carnal Christians. But true believers would not profess that they want to live that way. Jesus said, "So then, you will know them by their fruits" (Matt. 7:20).

Discernment Is a Gift from God

Jesus also said, "By this is My Father glorified, that you bear much fruit, and so prove to be My disciples" (John 15:8). That fruit should be evident in our lives, but it also includes the fruit of reproduction. False prophets, fake healers and bogus remedies will eventually be exposed over time. What the Church needs is the ability to discern. We can check their history, examine their faith and compare it with science, but that may not be enough. By human reason alone, we may not always be able to spot the counterfeit until it is too late. We may not know what is wrong, but the Holy Spirit will enable us to know that something is wrong. He is our first line of defense and we need to trust Him.

The interaction between God and Solomon is helpful in understanding discernment. David had died, and Solomon had taken his place as king of Israel. Solomon loved the Lord but, by his own admission, was too young and inexperienced to be the king.

> And now, O LORD my God, Thou has made Thy servant king in place of my father David, yet I am but a little child; I do not know how to go out or come in (1 Kings 3:7).

Before Solomon's admission, the Lord appeared to Solomon in a dream at night and said,

> Ask what you wish Me to give you (1 Kings 3:5).

With God's permission, Solomon asked, and the Lord responded.

> "Thy servant is in the midst of Thy people which Thou hast chosen, a great people who cannot be numbered or counted for multitude. So give Thy servant an understanding heart to judge Thy people to discern between good and evil. For who is able to judge this great people of Thine?" And it was pleasing in the sight of the Lord that

Solomon had asked this thing. And God said to him, "Because you have asked this thing and have not asked for yourself long life, nor have asked riches for yourself, nor have you asked for the life of your enemies, but have asked for yourself discernment to understand justice, behold, I have done according to your words. Behold, I have given you a wise and discerning heart, so that there has been no one like you before you, nor shall one like you arise after you" (1 Kings 3:8-12).

This passage reveals several key concepts about discernment.

God Gave Solomon the Ability to Discern Because of His Pure Motives

Solomon wasn't asking for personal gain or to have an advantage over his enemies. He was asking for the ability to discern good and evil, and God gave it to him. The ability to discern is dependent upon God, who looks at the heart. Although, if a person has the wrong motives for wanting to discern good and evil, this opens the door for Satan to attack.

I (Neil) noticed an undergraduate student who was following me around to various speaking engagements. After an evening service at a local church, she was shaking visibly. Learning that she was a student at our school, I asked her to stop by my office. At the same time she was also seeing one of our Christian counselors. When I asked her how that was going, she replied that her counseling sessions were like a game. She told me everything the counselor was going to do next. Realizing that she enjoyed playing mind games with her counselor, I challenged her, "You like doing that, don't you? You like the advantage it gives you over other people." As soon as I exposed the deception, an evil spirit manifested.

She believed God had given her a spiritual gift that gave her the ability to point out people's sins. She could walk on campus and say, "That person is struggling with sex; that person with alcohol, etc." As near as I could tell, she was right. This "gift from God" gave her the ability to know the evil in other people. However, when she found her freedom in Christ, the ability was gone. She was paying attention to an evil spirit that knew of the moral problems others were having. Her goal was to go into Christian counseling and use this gift to help people, while at the same time it was destroying her.

Spiritual Discernment Is Always on the Plane of Good and Evil

First Corinthians 12:10 reveals that the Holy Spirit enables all of us to discern between a good and evil spirit. I once worked with a young lady who was plagued with compulsive thoughts that contributed to her eating disorder. As she was going through the process of forgiving others, I sensed that it wasn't the girl talking anymore. There were two other people in the room observing the counseling process. "That's not her," I said. Nobody else discerned it, and they wondered how I knew. There was no objective way of knowing, but I discerned it was an evil spirit. The fact that my discernment was right became evident immediately. The expression on her face changed and a voice from her mouth said, "She will never forgive that person."

Spiritual discernment is primarily a function of the spirit, not the mind. I struggled with this concept for years, having been an ex-aerospace engineer. Discernment doesn't bypass the mind, nor does it replace the need to know the truth from God's Word. Rather, it builds upon the truth already known in our hearts. For example, there will be numerous occasions when we simply don't know or understand what is wrong from a rational perspective. Believers should be able to sense that a cult or occultic practitioner is not of the right spirit the moment they walk into the room. The Holy Spirit is letting us know that something is wrong. It's like an alarm going off. Our minds ask for objectivity. We want to know what's wrong, but the Holy Spirit is only alerting us that something is wrong. The Holy Spirit's signal is our first line of defense, which functions like an early warning system.

Let me illustrate this point by showing how discernment works for a parent with children at home (many years ago for me). Suppose my son comes home, and I sense something is wrong. I ask him, "What's wrong, Karl?" He says, "Nothing!" Again I ask him what's wrong, and again he claims nothing is wrong. However, my "buzzer" goes off, because I discern that something is wrong. In order to be objective, I guess what it is (Is that being objective?)! "Have you been doing such and such again?" If I guess wrong (and I probably will), I will blow the discernment, which leads to my son stalking into his room, mad at me, for falsely charging him.

So what should I do? Just share the discernment. "Karl, something is wrong!" "No, Dad, nothing's wrong!" "Karl, I know something is wrong!" He shrugs his shoulders and goes to his room. Is that it? Of course not! The Holy Spirit enables me to discern, but He is also convicting him of sin. What is happening in his room? Conviction! And he is probably thinking, *Dad knows!*

There Is Nothing Magical About Discernment and It Is Not Human Intuition Either

It only makes sense that the Holy Spirit in our lives is going to warn us against the presence of an evil spirit. "You cannot drink the cup of the Lord and the cup of demons; you cannot partake of the table of the Lord and the table of demons" (1 Cor. 10:21). The Holy Spirit does not remain passive in the face of adversity.

> For though by this time you ought to be teachers, you have need again for someone to teach you the elementary principles of the oracles of God, and you have come to need milk and not solid food. For everyone who partakes only of milk is not accustomed to the word of righteousness, for he is a babe. But solid food is for the mature, who because of practice have their senses trained to discern good and evil. Therefore leaving the elementary teaching about the Christ, let us press on to maturity, not laying again a foundation of repentance from dead works and of faith toward God, of instruction about washings, and laying on of hands, and the resurrection of the dead, and eternal judgment (Heb. 5:12—6:2).

What the writer identifies as elementary teaching is heavy theology for most people. A good systematic theology is the foundation upon which we build our lives, and it is to our faith-filled walk with God what our skeleton is to our body. Faith holds us together and keeps us in the right form. Good doctrine is never an end in itself. True doctrine governs our relationship with God and man. Many Christians aren't ready for solid food, because they haven't had their senses trained to discern good and evil. Their relationship to God is only theological and not personal. But those accustomed to the Word of righteousness are sensitive to the leading of the Holy Spirit.

WHAT ARE FOUR POSSIBLE SIGNS OF A DECEIVED CHRISTIAN?

One of the biggest problems we see is that deceived people are not aware that they are deceived. Therefore, we conclude this chapter by offering four standards by which we can test and check the spirit.

1. **Relationship with God.** Are you or the person you are concerned about doing well spiritually and growing in your relationship with God? Or is there a spiritual coldness, a sense of estrangement from God or a loss of interest or joy? The Holy Spirit bears witness with our spirit that we are children of God, which enables us to commune with our heavenly Father, filling us with joy and peace (see Rom. 8:16). The first red flag that the Holy Spirit is not in control is when there's a loss of intimacy with the Father and the joy and peace that naturally accompany Him (see Gen. 3:8-10; Gal. 5:22-23).

2. **Relationship with church leadership.** Christ, the head of the Church, has established pastors and elders as spiritual shepherds over His flock. They are to feed the flock and humbly lead and protect (see 1 Pet. 5:1-8). Do you sense a rebellious spirit? Are you listening to, respecting and honoring your church leadership? Or are you ignoring, avoiding or resisting? "Obey them that have the rule over you, and submit yourselves: for they watch for your souls, as they that must give account, that they may do it with joy, and not with grief: for that is unprofitable for you" (Heb. 13:17, *KJV*).

3. **Relationship with the Body of Christ.** Do you have close fellowship with your church body? Having no accountability with your brothers and sisters in Christ leaves you vulnerable. A lion or pack of wolves isolates a vulnerable sheep from the rest of the flock prior to devouring it. Similarly, when a Christian becomes isolated from the Body of Christ, it is evident that the adversary (who is likened to both a lion and wolf) is involved.

4. **Physical health.** Is your physical health improving or is it deteriorating? A person entrapped in a deceptive health practice will truly believe that they are being helped by it. And yet, it is an illusion, because overall, from an objective standpoint, their health is sliding downhill.

RALPH AND AMY'S APPLICATION #5

Amy's doctor used a combination of computerized electrical testing of meridian points along with muscle testing to determine her disease and treatment program (see chapter 2). When he needed to know the dosage to give her, the doctor asked Amy's body to tell him. Silently he inquired, "Do you need two pills?" If the answer was yes, her body told him so by her arm becoming strong. If the answer was no, she tested weak.

As we proposed earlier in this chapter, there appears to be no purely physical reason for how a body could give an answer to a question verbally presented to it. Using arm strength as a signal to represent a body's answer to a verbal question appears to be no different in principle than using a pendulum to obtain information from the immaterial realm. Both appear to be divination, and, if so, the spirit involved is not the Holy Spirit. (Some with prior involvement in the New Age movement say questions addressed in these types of scenarios are to a spirit guide.) When Ralph and Amy recognized this serious possibility, they decided to renounce the activity and no longer pursue treatment with this particular practitioner. They determined that despite the fact that this chiropractor was thought to be a Christian, his professional approach appeared incompatible with biblical faith.

In Conclusion

We must learn to exercise spiritual discernment. Is the supernatural involved? If yes, is it the Holy Spirit or another spirit? If it is a spirit other than the Holy Spirit, it is an illusion, a masquerading counterfeit. Absolute truth will bear up under testing, so check the spirit and it will reveal itself.

CHAPTER EIGHT

ASSUMING RESPONSIBILITY FOR OUR OWN HEALTH

There can be no stable and balanced development of the mind apart from the assumption of responsibility.

JOHN DEWEY

Man must cease attributing his problems to his environment, and learn again to exercise his will—his personal responsibility in the realm of faith and morals.

ALBERT SCHWEITZER

As commander of the Syrian army, Naaman was used to being in the midst of danger. A brave and seasoned warrior, he had led numerous successful campaigns during his military career. But all of his success, military prowess and high esteem in which even the king held him were brought to naught by a devastating diagnosis of leprosy.

Certainly a man of his stature and prominence would have access to the best medical care in the world at that time and, thereby, obtain a cure for this disease, which was equivalent to a death sentence. But such was not to be the case. Every doctor he had consulted with and every treatment he tried had failed.

One day, a captured Hebrew slave girl told him about a man of God back in her homeland who had done great miracles. She was confident that this prophet could cure Naaman's leprosy. Perhaps in desperation, the king of Syria sent Naaman to Israel, along with a letter and a large fortune to seek the favor of this great prophet.

But Naaman did not even receive the dignity of a personal greeting. Before he arrived at the home of Elisha, a message was sent to him from the prophet by way of a servant. He was told to take a bath in the Jordan River seven times. If he did so his leprosy would be cleansed (see 2 Kings 5:10).

The Jordan River? Why, there were better rivers back home in Syria! No way, was Naaman's response. Deeply offended, he "went away in a rage" (v. 12). But his servants appealed to him and begged him to reconsider. So Naaman begrudgingly went to the Jordan. After bathing himself a seventh time, his skin was restored to that "of a little child" (v. 14).

Naaman learned a very important principle. God, in His wisdom and love, deals individually with each one of us according to our needs as He sees them. Certainly, bathing in the dirty Jordan River was not a legitimate medical treatment for leprosy, either then or now. Furthermore, there is nothing in Scripture to indicate that this procedure will cure someone with leprosy. But that is not the point. The point is that God saw not only Naaman's need for physical healing but also his heart.

God Knows Our Real Need

First of all, God saw Naaman's pride, which almost cost him God's blessing. Secondly, God saw that Naaman had a distorted perception of Him and His grace. Naaman thought God's grace could be earned. He wanted to pay Elisha for his services, which he probably had to do to succor his pagan gods back home. But Elisha would take no payment; he knew that the grace of God is not for sale.

God designed a specific treatment to meet not only Naaman's physical need but also his spiritual needs. As a result, Naaman not only was healed of leprosy, but also he came to believe and trust in the true and living God.[1]

We Need to Desire Wellness

The story of Naaman tells us something else about being healed: We need to truly desire healing, enough that we are willing to do whatever God asks of us.

John records the story of a man who was sick for 38 years. He was lying by a pool near Bethesda, hoping that he would be the first to take the plunge, when an angel stirred the waters. Jesus asked him, "Do you wish to get well?" (John 5:6). Instead of answering the question, the man offered an excuse, exhibiting no faith in God. There was no one to put him in the water (see v. 7). But the Lord's sovereignty healed him, and the man thanked Jesus not with gracious praise and thanksgiving but by telling the Jews that Jesus had healed him on the Sabbath, leading to more persecution for Jesus (see vv. 15-16). The man really didn't want to get well, and there are many people like him today. Illnesses can attract a lot of attention and provide excuses for people to not live a responsible life. Therefore, we have to ask the hard question: Do you wish to get well?

DECISIONS ARE THE PATIENT'S RESPONSIBILITY

If you desire to live a life of wellness, then you should be willing to take whatever steps are necessary in order to get or stay well. This may include changing your diet, exercising, repenting and assuming responsibility for your own health. Nobody else can do that for you. We can't eat for you, exercise for you or make the crucial decisions that you must make concerning your life. We will never see good physical, mental, emotional and spiritual health in our churches unless people realize that to have such is their responsibility. We can't do your praying for you, believe for you, repent for you or forgive others for you, and we love you enough to tell you that. Elisha did not go to the Jordan and bathe there on Naaman's behalf. Naaman had to do it if he was ever going to experience the healing that he desired and God was offering.

James 5:13-16—the only place in the Epistles that tells us what to do if we are sick—begins by instructing the one who is suffering to pray. While nobody else can do your praying for you, we do believe in intercessory prayer, but not to replace your responsibility to pray. If you had two boys and the younger brother kept asking the older brother to ask you for something on his behalf, what would you do as a parent? Wouldn't you send that older brother back and have him tell his younger brother that he needs to talk to you himself? Would you accept a secondhand relationship with your own son? God doesn't either. In fact, you can't have a secondhand relationship with God. Jesus is the only intermediary between God and His children—you must have a personal, one-on-one relationship with Him.

James also instructs the person who is sick to take the initiative to "call the elders of the church" and request prayer (v. 14). God makes it our responsibility to seek His healing with the help of other believers. This eliminates the problem of pride. James then instructs the sick person to confess his or her sins (see v. 16). Only then do the prayers of another righteous person become effective (see v. 16). However, it is not right to expect the prayer of others to bring healing to your body if you are living in sin. As we discussed in chapter 4, some physical illnesses (including what we call the psychosomatic illnesses) are due to sin. This is probably what James is alluding to in this passage.

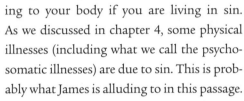
To be spiritually mature, you have to know God's truth and live accordingly by faith with the power of the Holy Spirit.

Good health is not contagious. You can sit by a healthy person for years, but it will not have any positive impact on your health. If you wanted to be healthy like that person, you would have to learn what they believe and live accordingly by faith. The same is true spiritually. Sitting by a mature person will not make you more spiritual. There is no such thing as spiritual or physical osmosis. To be spiritually mature, you have to know God's truth and live accordingly by faith with the power of the Holy Spirit.

WE NEED TO LISTEN TO THE HOLY SPIRIT

The story of Naaman also illustrates the importance of being led by the Holy Spirit. It is not uncommon for mature Christians, who normally seek God for direction in every area of their lives, to turn off their "spiritual ears" when they go into a doctor's office. Instead of trusting their discernment, they do whatever their physician says. King Asa made that mistake. Scripture says that though his disease was "exceeding great: yet in his disease he sought not to the LORD, but to the physicians" (2 Chron. 16:12, *KJV*). Countless times, after giving patients their medical options and asking them for their decision, their response to me (Michael) has been something akin to, "You're the doctor. You decide."

I decide? Since when did God give me the authority to make health-care decisions in someone else's life? He didn't give me (or any other physician) that authority, but I do have the responsibility to inform my patients of my professional opinion based on my knowledge of medicine and God's Word. Unfortunately, there are some physicians who will make those decisions for you, and they may become defensive if you question their decision or seek a second opinion. In some cases, patients can feel intimidated by the diplomas on the wall and simply yield to the physician's will. But if things go wrong, malpractice suits usually follow. Living outside your realm of responsibility inevitably exposes you to greater liability.

Biblically speaking, the responsibility for medical decisions rests squarely on the shoulders of the patient (or, especially in the case of children, on the parents). Therefore, it is imperative that patients are spiritually discerning and fully informed.

At 40 years of age, Pastor Larry Cornett suddenly developed severe neck pain radiating into his left arm. After failing to respond to chiropractic therapy, an MRI scan revealed two herniated disks in his neck. He was promptly referred to a neurosurgeon. After taking one look at his scan, the neurosurgeon told the young pastor that surgery was needed within two weeks if he was to preserve the use of his left arm. The surgical approach would be from the front, going through the throat, to the spinal column. There was a 20 percent risk of permanent damage to the vocal cords.

Despite the pressure placed upon him by his neurosurgeon, Pastor Cornett insisted on prayerfully seeking the Lord for His direction. The more he prayed, the less peace he had about the operation. Then through a mutual acquaintance, he heard of an injection procedure that could possibly resolve his condition and spare him of the need for surgery. He was eventually referred to my office where a simple, inexpensive injection treatment (known as prolotherapy) corrected his condition. That was 10 years ago. Pastor Cornett has yet to need that surgery. In addition, God used His "divine appointment" between Pastor Cornett and me to answer the prayers of my wife and me, leading our family to move to Cincinnati where Larry Cornett is now our pastor.

Doctors should never attempt to play the role of God. Neither should they be the final authority in a patient's life. But they do provide an essential service to the community and deserve our respect. I had a patient who I believed, like Pastor Cornett, could avoid back surgery if he opted for prolotherapy. Instead, he chose surgery, because he was intimidated by his doctor and he didn't want to offend him. It would have been good at the time for him to heed to Proverbs 29:25:

> The fear of man brings a snare, but he who trusts in the Lord will be exalted.

WE NEED TO DISCERN GOD'S WILL

Alice had a burden of a different sort. She had the responsibility of caring for her young teenage son who had been afflicted since birth with a potentially fatal disease. During one of his many hospitalizations, his central IV line, by which he received his daily feedings, became infected. It was obvious that the contaminated catheter needed to be replaced. Her son's new physicians wanted to take him to the operating room and do the procedure under general anesthesia.

 Doctors should never attempt to play the role of God. Neither should they be the final authority in a patient's life. But they do provide an essential service to the community and deserve our respect.

This seemed odd to Alice, since throughout the first several years of his life, central lines had always been replaced under local anesthesia, sparing the risk of using mechanical ventilation and inhalation drugs. However, intimidated by the unfamiliar doctors in this expert treatment facility, Alice quietly consented to the procedure despite her lack of peace.

Unfortunately, while in the operating room, the ventilator pressure ruptured one of her son's lungs. As a result, he was forced to remain paralyzed and on a breathing machine for several weeks until it healed. I (Michael) recall speaking with Alice on the phone shortly after the event. I remember her asking me, "Do you think my lack of peace was the Holy Spirit trying to caution me to insist on local anesthesia?" If our hearts are filled with fear, or we are feeling pressured, it becomes more difficult to discern God's guidance. We need to pause and, if at all possible, get alone with God and seek His guidance. We could spare ourselves much grief by doing this.[2]

WE NEED TO LIVE IN ACCORDANCE WITH OUR MEASURE OF FAITH

As we learned earlier from Naaman's story, God knows each one of us and understands our unique needs. This is especially true in regard to our level of faith and why He may direct one person in one way and someone else in another, even if they are two people with the same diagnosis. In order to explain the unique role that faith plays, we will use the following illustration.

Suppose you were a missionary in China and came down with symptoms of a cold that you couldn't seem to get over. What if you went to a doctor who came highly recommended and was an expert in the area of herbs? Let's say that you had a problem with nasal congestion and cough, and so he prescribed a Chinese herbal concoction known as Ma Huang Tang.

When you asked him how the remedy worked, he explained that you had "encountered a wind cold evil" and were displaying a "Tai Yang stage pattern." The four substances in the concoction were designed to be acrid and warm and promote sweating, dispel cold and "resolve the surface."[3]

Obviously, as a Westerner, this explanation would not make much sense to you. Perhaps you may recognize the explanation to be rooted in Taoism. As a Christian, you have at least two possible responses in this situation.

1. Leave the doctor's office and determine not to follow his advice, since the philosophy behind his practice and advice is obviously contrary to your Christian faith. Furthermore, you may feel the need to abstain from following his advice because you publicly represent the Christian faith, and you are concerned that your participation might be perceived as an endorsement of his pagan belief system.

2. You could choose to believe that the Chinese people may have learned good things about herbs over the centuries and decide to follow the doctor's advice, but still reject his Taoist views. In this case, you accept the fact that God is the one who made the herbs for their medicinal value, but you do not accept the Taoist explanation as to why they work. With a little research, you discover that Ma Huang Tang is a natural source for ephedra. Assuming that the herb helped your symptoms, you might attribute the benefit not to the

balancing of yin and yang, but to the fact that ephedra stimulates beta receptors in the smooth muscle of blood vessels, causing them to constrict and, thereby, act as a decongestant.

The direction you choose depends upon your personal faith, your understanding of science and the leading of the Holy Spirit. The issues addressed in the above scenario are not uncommon, and you don't have to be missionaries in China to encounter them. They are happening with increasing frequency in the western hemisphere.

WE NEED TO FOLLOW BIBLICAL ABSOLUTES

In Scripture, there are teachings, such as the problem of eating or not eating meat that was sacrificed to idols, and whether or not the Israelites should continue the kosher traditions of the Jewish community, which are classified as disputable matters. Disputable matters are not fundamental to the Christian faith and are usually matters in which individual Christians may differ in opinion without impacting their salvation. Most, if not at all, health-care issues are disputable matters. They are matters of preference and should never be allowed to divide our fellowship with other believers. Paul addresses disputable matters quite extensively in Romans 14–15. The following three principles summarize how we should respond to disputable matters:

1. Whatever you do, do it unto God out of love for Him. Be fully convinced of the truth in your own minds (see Rom. 14:5-8,22-23).
2. Live freely according to your preferences, but don't judge others on their matters of preference (see Rom. 14:4-22).
3. Walk in genuine love for others and do not exercise your freedom at their expense (see Rom. 14:15-21; 15:1-8).

APPLICATION

So how does one apply these concepts to medicine and health? First, we should strive for balance. Heresy almost never begins with blatant error; it begins with truth out of balance. If you believe everything the clerks at your health-food store say, you may need a truck to buy all the supplements they recommend. If you believe everything your fitness gurus say, you may be exercising 20 hours a day. If you believe everything your dermatologists say, you will never go out in the sun again. If you believe everything your dieticians say, you will never enjoy another meal. The key: Listen and find the right balance for you.

Second, do all things in moderation, and be less rigid and more flexible with yourself and others. The moral parameters of God allow us room to exercise our preferences. Live under the grace of God and enjoy life. This is what the Christian life is supposed to be. Instead of a long list of rigid laws that dictate our daily behavior, God has put His Spirit within us. He will guide us into all truth, enabling us to live a liberated life in Christ, but not at the expense of others. As with Naaman, God knows us individually. He understands our individual needs and will direct our steps accordingly.

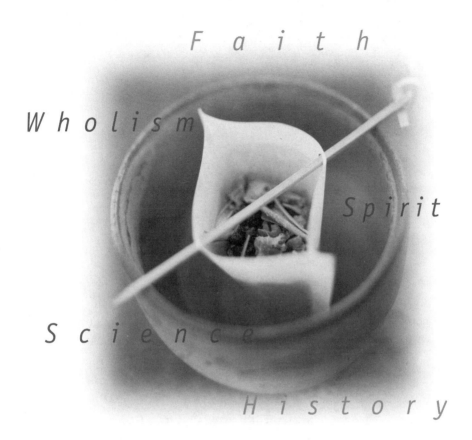

Faith

Wholism

Spirit

Science

History

PART 2

EVALUATING MEDICAL SYSTEMS

CHAPTER NINE

AYURVEDA

Ayur-Ved is the world's original system of health care.

FUNDAMENTALS OF MAHARISHI AYUR-VED

My (Michael's) family does not have a reputation for producing great out-doorsmen. I recall one of our typical fishing outings as a youth. My father, brothers and I went out on a rowboat on Lake Minnetonka, near Minneapolis. Before long, two of us hooked what we thought were large northern pikes. After a great battle lasting several minutes, my father suggested the possibility that we had caught each other's lines rather than two large fish. To our chagrin, we discovered that he was right. Reeling our lines into the boat revealed a snarled mess that, at first glance, looked impossible to untangle.

A similar feeling to the one I felt on the boat that day happened when I observed the conglomeration of history and ideas patched together into what are known as Hinduism and Ayurveda (ay-yoor-va-duh). These two traditions do not represent one clear development of thought over the course of time. Instead, it seems that the Hindu leaders repeatedly added any new concept that was to their liking—regardless of its compatibility with prior convention—to their belief systems.

If we hold to the rules of logic, then every proponent of Ayurveda is by def-inition completely out of step with divine revelation and Jesus, who said, "I am the way, and the truth, and the life" (John 14:6). Christianity has always held that the Bible is the sole source for faith and practice. Once man abandons absolute truth, it is impossible to explain life without confusion and self-contradiction. Only in Christ "are hidden *all* the treasures of wisdom and knowledge" (Col. 2:3, emphasis added). However, investing a small amount of time in grasping a few major concepts of Ayurveda will reap huge dividends in understanding what is happening in our medical world today.

EVALUATING THROUGH THE GRID OF HISTORY

In a 1995 publication entitled *Fundamentals of Maharishi Ayur-Ved,* the authors make an incredible assertion: "Historically, Ayur-Ved is the world's original system of health care. It is the basis of Greek medicine, which is the root of much of Western medicine."[1] Their claim is not far-fetched. Ayurvedic concepts form the basis of not only many other energy-based medical approaches, including traditional Chinese medicine (TCM), but the concepts also serve as the philosophical roots of modern medicine. Because of Ayurveda's roots, we begin by evaluating it first.

Ayurveda is a Sanskrit (the ancient language of India) compound name of two words, *ayus* meaning "life" and *veda* meaning "knowledge."[2] It is a non-Christian holistic system that not only encompasses medicine but also an entire approach to life. It traces its origins to the Vedas—ancient religious manuscripts written somewhere between 1500 B.C. and 500 B.C., which preceded the development of Hinduism.[3] Ayurveda is the quadrant of the Vedas that deals with physical healing, diet, herbs and massage. The central purpose of Ayurveda is to attain optimum physical well-being so that the individual is free to pursue "the path of Yoga" (i.e., the right path) unencumbered by health concerns.[4]

Over the centuries, significant additions were made to Ayurveda, including examination of the urine and the radial pulse in the wrist (this concept is also prominent in TCM).[5] However, during the period in which India was ruled by foreign power, classical Ayurveda was all but discarded. Its recent resurrection is attributed to the influence of Maharishi Mahesh Yogi, the father of the transcendental meditation (TM) movement in America, and to a receptive audience in the West.[6] While Ayurveda has been practiced by a small minority of physicians in the West, its popularity has risen in recent years due to the success of its most public representative Deepak Chopra, M.D. His goal is that Ayurveda eventually become part of mainstream medical education in the West.[7]

EVALUATING THROUGH THE GRID OF FAITH

Every pagan nation has its gods. India has millions of deities. Belief in these deities plays a significant role in the everyday life of the Hindu, and they are sought after by the sick for healing. However, we will dismiss them from our consideration at this point, since it is the pantheistic concepts from the Vedas that prevail in Ayurveda. The dominant worldview in India is pantheism, which is a belief that all is god. The philosophy of pantheism exchanges a personal God for impersonal energy.

> The goal of Ayurveda is for each individual to develop the highest level of consciousness and, thereby, attain union with universal intelligence and with one another.

In the Western scientific model of medicine, the basis for understanding physical health is primarily rooted in the physical or material realm. With the exception of some Christian doctors and nurses, people are understood to be biological machines, and diseases are treated with physical agents such as medication, surgery, diet, physical therapy, etc. In the Western scientific worldview, people are composed of solid miniature bits of matter.

In stark contrast, Ayurveda believes that the basis of life and health is rooted in the nonmaterial realm—in a field of energy—known as *prana*.[8] Citing quantum physics as its proof, Ayurvedic proponents explain that the smallest particles in the universe, electrons and protons, are not solid and material but rather immaterial. These discrete particles make up a giant waveform energy field known as a force field or superfield.

This fundamental energy field is not in a state of disarray. Instead, it vibrates at a uniform frequency or in a wavelike motion. According to this belief, all other matter (including human beings) have at their core a nonmaterial waveform, which is derived from this underlying energy field. Most important, this immaterial energy field is conceived of as a field of "pure intelligence."

All the order and intelligence of the laws of nature arise from this one fundamental, nonmaterial field, as does all matter. Not only are particles really just waves; those waves ultimately are made of an underlying field, as ocean waves are made of ocean water. This field is one of pure intelligence, having the attributes that we associate with consciousness.[9]

According to this paradigm, a person gets sick because he or she loses his or her connection to (or actually his or her memory of) this field of consciousness or pure intelligence. Therefore, someone can only get well by "restoring one's conscious connection to (or memory of) this innermost core of one's being and experience."[10]

Thus, the goal of Ayurveda is for each individual to develop the highest level of consciousness and, thereby, attain union with universal intelligence and with one another. This is very similar to the concept of *moksa* in Hinduism, Ayurveda's next-of-kin that is best known for its belief in reincarnation and *karma*. Karma predetermines a person's birth, place in society, health and length of life on the basis of how well he or she performs in a previous life. In moksa, the highest aim of life is liberation from the cycle of birth, suffering and rebirth. This is principally accomplished by means of higher and higher meditative states until one achieves union with the divine or ultimate consciousness.[11]

Liberation is release from this cycle of rebirth. It is typically to be achieved by working out those karmic residues which have already begun to mature, as well as by following certain practices to ensure that no further residues are produced to cause future rebirths. The practices by which one can achieve this are frequently termed yoga, and the theory of liberation is the core of Indian philosophy.[12]

EVALUATING THROUGH THE WHOLISTIC GRID

In one sense, Ayurveda is wholistic, and that is why many people frustrated with the purely biomedical model of Western medicine are attracted to it. However, their perception of reality matches neither natural or spiritual law as created and governed by God. In Ayurveda, universal prana energy (cosmic consciousness) is believed to give rise to five basic elements or principles: earth, air, fire, water and ether. These elements interact with one another to comprise all physical matter. This concept dates back over 2,500 years, prior to the discovery of basic chemistry and physics principles.[13] In the human body, these five elements are further organized into three broader principles or elements known as *doshas*. The three doshas are *vata* (air and ether), *pitta* (fire and water, manifesting as bile) and *kapha* (earth and water, manifesting as phlegm).[14]

Determine Your Dosha Type

According to Ayurveda, each individual is born with a predetermined combination of the doshas. A person may have a natural predisposition toward one of them; however, the doshas must be in harmony with one another in order for there to be optimum health. When imbalance occurs, sickness ensues. In other words, "all disease results from a disruption of the natural balance of the doshas."[15] In fact, diseases are classified according to what dosha predisposition they represent.[16] Recall that Maharishi Ayurveda teaches that all disease is secondary to losing one's connection to (or memory of) a universal intelligence or energy field. In Ayurveda, energy and matter are all one. As we will see in the next chapter, the Greeks brought the concept of dosha balance into Western medicine, where the doshas became known as *humors*.

Additionally, the three doshas are linked with the seasons of the year, the time of day, the weather, certain foods and personality types. Therefore, Ayurveda emphasizes the need for individuals to maintain balance by living in harmony with their particular dosha and the parameters that it dictates, such as the type of food to eat, the daily routine to follow and the behavior to exemplify.[17]

Determine Your Disease Type

Imbalance in the doshas can occur for a variety of reasons, including unhealthy mental or emotional patterns, poor diet, inadequate rest, stress, etc. This disharmony results in a weakening of the body's resistance to disease and a buildup of toxins, referred to as *ama*.[18] When sickness develops, the Ayurvedic practitioner's first goal is to bring the doshas back into balance. In order to accomplish this, the practitioner must first determine the patient's dosha type. He or she does this by considering the patient's body habitus, personality type and behavior.

The next step is for the practitioner to determine the nature of their patient's illness. He or she assesses the patient's radial artery pulse with three fingers to determine the presence of a dosha imbalance. A pulse pattern characteristic of a snake (at the index finger) indicates vata predisposition, while that of a frog (at the middle finger) indicates pitta and that of a swan (at the ring finger) confirms kapha. Another examination is made of external features such as the tongue, nails and skin, in addition to the urine.[19]

Determine Your Treatment

Once the dosha and the nature of the disease have been determined, treatment is initiated to restore balance. This is accomplished through a variety of means.

1. **Purification therapy**. This involves a five-step process to rid the body of toxins (ama) and any excess dosha. Excess of bile (pitta) is removed by giving the patient an emetic to make him vomit. Purgatives are used to remove an abundance of phlegm (kapha). Enemas cause the body to expel excess air (vata). Smoke inhalation or nasal drops are given to rid the head of excess dosha, and leeches, or bloodletting, are applied to purify the blood.
2. **Remedies**. These are historically herbal preparations. However, according to one source, "75 percent of the preparations recommended by Ayurvedic practitioners are modern (present-day) pharmaceutical drugs."[20]
3. **Diet.** Practitioners usually recommend a vegetarian diet. Digestion is emphasized.
4. **Miscellaneous.** Massage with sesame oil is another popular treatment. It removes toxins from the body.

Determine Your Plan for Prevention

Once health is restored, Ayurveda seeks to maintain optimum health through attaining and maintaining optimum balance in the person's material being (physical body) and immaterial being (i.e., spiritual or energy). This is accomplished principally through the following steps:[21]

1. Develop higher states of consciousness in order to "reconnect" and maintain union with universal intelligence. This is accomplished primarily through transcendental meditation (TM) and yoga. In Hinduism, the ultimate goal of these activities is liberation from karma.[22]

"Yoga," a Sanskrit word generally meaning "union," refers to a method of gaining release from the bondage of karma and rebirth, which constitutes the highest aim for most Hindus, Buddhists and Jains.

Yoga teaches breath control and postures, which are designed to allow adepts to concentrate without having their minds distracted by extraneous things. By concentrating on progressively more abstract concepts, yogis achieve higher and higher meditative states, culminating in a contentless trance (nirvikalpaka samadhi) that constitutes liberation. Yogis in more advanced stages of this process are said to be endowed with remarkable powers (siddhis), such as special capacities for sight, levitation and projection of their minds into other bodies.[23]

2. Dietary choices and daily schedules designed to coincide with the person's dosha type.
3. Massage with sesame oil stimulates the flow of energy at specific *marma* points (similar to Chinese acupuncture points), which rebalance doshas and move toxins so that they are eliminated by the body.
4. Intestinal cleansing procedures done periodically on a preventative basis.[24]

EVALUATING THROUGH THE GRID OF SCIENCE

Living a balanced life and employing a nutritious diet have tremendous health benefits. However, these are not unique to Ayurveda. They are common to many medical paradigms and consistent with living in harmony with God's natural and spiritual laws. However, we have been able to find very little credible scientific data to indicate that Ayurveda, in general, is effective in the treatment of disease. The basis given for Ayurveda is largely theoretical (i.e., just ideas) or anecdotal (individual testimonies).[25] Most Ayurvedic herbal remedies have not undergone scientific scrutiny. While a few preparations have shown some promise, most are untested. Furthermore, according to a leading authority on Ayurveda, "The majority of Ayurvedic formulations on the [Western] market are either spurious, adulterated or misbranded."[26]

On the other hand, yoga has demonstrated improvement in people's physical fitness and flexibility, while also relieving stress and chronic pain.[27] In a 1998 study out of the University of Pennsylvania School of Medicine, yoga was found to be somewhat more helpful than standard wrist splinting in reducing pain and improving grip strength in patients suffering from carpal tunnel syndrome (CTS). Twenty-two people received one to one and one-half hours of instruction, twice weekly, by a yoga instructor who focused on taking each upper body joint through its full range of motion with strengthening, stretching and balancing. Each session was concluded with a relaxation phase.[28] One has to wonder if physical therapy of the wrists and arms—rather than just splinting—would have accomplished the same as the yoga sessions but without the spiritual component.

Yoga involves not only physical movement and posturing but also meditation. The potential health benefits of yoga and TM are a reduction of stress, blood pressure, anxiety and pain.[29] These benefits appear to directly affect the ability of those practicing meditation to obtain a state of true relaxation. Apparently, the recitation of yoga mantras at a consistent rate of six times per minute assists the body in slowing breathing to a rate of six breaths per minute, which reinforces basic healthy autonomic control patterns over the heart. Interestingly, an Italian study demonstrated that the same physiologic effects were accomplished when the rosary was prayed (chanted) at the same six-times-per-minute rate.[30]

Chanting mantras or rosary prayers at a timed rate is not the only means by which favorable cardiac electrical patterns can be consciously induced. Studies have shown that positive emotional states—feelings of compassion, love or gratefulness—induce similar benefits in heart rate variability (HRV) patterns. HRV measures the influence of the autonomic system's control over the heart and is considered by some as the best single test available to predict risk of sudden cardiac death. Theoretically then, as with relaxation, when people are experiencing these positive emotional states, their risk of heart attack is significantly reduced. However, we do not know this for fact. Additionally, we are unaware of any data that shows that relaxation—by meditation or yoga—actually reduces the incidence of disease.

The Big Picture

Rather than a further detailed look at scientific studies, perhaps it would be most helpful to back up a little and look at the big picture. Ayurveda is a system of medicine that has been in place for at least 2,500 years. If it were such a superior approach to medicine, would it not have produced those results in its mother country, and would not the claims of its adherents have been validated long before now?

The fact remains that on more than one occasion in the past, Ayurveda's concepts have been adopted by other medical systems but with disastrous results. This will become particularly evident when we look at the history of Western allopathic medicine. Only when allopathy abandoned the Ayurvedic roots—which had been passed on to it through the Greeks—that shackled it for 2,300 years did it finally see a system develop that was of some objective value in combating disease (see chapter 10 on allopathic medicine). As with many alternative paradigms being offered today, Ayurveda is lauded not because there is great evidence of its effectiveness, but because it is different than established medicine.

Recall the pattern set forth in the first three chapters of this book. The Maharishi Yogi, TM, yoga and Ayurveda came into the U.S. in the 1970s, in the wake of the 1960s cultural revolution. Looking for fresh certainties, our culture is turning to the past, to ancient healing paradigms, because when on this side of a revolution, the distant past always seems more stable.

EVALUATING THROUGH THE GRID OF SPIRITUAL DISCERNMENT

Ayurveda's greatest strength—its ability through meditation to induce a complete state of relaxation—is Christianity's greatest spiritual threat. Indeed, its own adherents claim that the reason for TM's superiority over other relaxation techniques is that in TM one experiences "the fourth state of consciousness" (referred to as transcendental consciousness), in which enlightenment or unification with "pure intelligence" occurs.[31] To achieve this state, one must bypass the mind and pursue truth directly. This is in direct contradiction to Christianity. God never bypasses our minds; He works through them. In fact, we are transformed by the renewing of our minds (see Rom. 12:2). We, as believers, are most spiritually vulnerable when we reach a passive state of mind. That is one reason why we are instructed by Jesus not to pray in vain repetitions. Mindlessly repeating a mantra for 20 minutes will produce a dull state of the mind, and that is the intended purpose for TM and other transcendental exercises. But in Christ, He wants our minds fresh and alive—always ready for His calling.

From a biblical and scientific standpoint, this transcendental state may come at a price. Some reports indicate that almost half of active TM trainers report "episodes of anxiety, depression, confusion, frustration . . . mental and physical tension . . . and antisocial behavior."[32] Clearly, with a stated goal of removing one's mind from attachment to physical reality and its problems, yogis are attempting to contact that which is supernatural or immaterial. Yogis claim that with higher and higher meditative states,

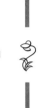

We, as believers, are most spiritually vulnerable when we reach a passive state of mind.

they are able to levitate and project their minds into others' bodies—the psychic realm is being breached.[33] In scriptural terms, this is the realm of the demonic.

Biblical Analysis

Meditation is a Christian discipline, but it always has an object. Meditation, like faith, is only validated by its object. The critical question is not whether you believe, but what or who you believe in. The same is true for meditation. If you meditate on nothing, it will have disastrous results. Scripture clearly instructs us to meditate on God's word.

> Blessed is the man . . . [whose] delight is in the law of the LORD; and in his law doth he meditate day and night (Ps. 1:1-2, *KJV*).

> My eyes anticipate the night watches, that I may meditate on Thy word (Ps. 119:148).

> My meditation of him shall be sweet: I will be glad in the LORD (Ps. 104:34, *KJV*).

> I remember the days of old; I meditate on all thy works; I muse on the work of thy hands (Ps. 143:5, *KJV*).

Many Christians have not disciplined themselves to meditate on God's Word. Therefore, they do not experience the full spiritual and physical benefit of doing so. The concept of meditation in the Hebrew paints a picture of sheep chewing cud. When sheep graze, the food is not swallowed whole and then passed through the body. Instead, it is chewed thoroughly and then swallowed. It then travels to one of several stomach chambers where it is acted upon by enzymes and regurgitated back to the mouth, where it is chewed once again. Only with repeated swallowing and rechewing are the most valuable nutritional components (such as protein) gleaned from the food.[34]

So it is with God's Word. If it is quickly read and then forgotten for the rest of the day, its value to the believer is minimal.

> For if any be a hearer of the word, and not a doer, he is like unto a man beholding his natural face in a glass: For he beholdeth himself, and goeth his way, and straightway forgetteth what manner of man he was (Jas. 1:23-24, *KJV*).

But when the truth is understood and it enters our heart, the result is personal transformation and better physical, mental, emotional and spiritual health.

If we approached biblical meditation with the same intensity that is ascribed to those who practice TM, it would produce greater results, since the focus is upon God and His truth rather than on a quantum force field with all the inherent spiritual dangers. (See chapter 20 for a biblical analysis of thought, meditation, mind-body and New Age medicine.)

Ayurveda, Hinduism and Christianity Parallels and Distinctions

There are several interesting parallels in Ayurveda and Hinduism to Christian thought, but each has critically important distinctions.

1. The first cause of and sustainer of the universe is immaterial. But instead of impersonal energy or a force field, God is a personal being, a Spirit with personhood.

   > In the beginning God created the heaven and the earth. And the earth was without form, and void; and darkness was upon the face of the deep. And the spirit of God moved upon the face of the waters (Gen. 1:1-2, *KJV*).

God is a Spirit: and they that worship him must worship him in spirit and in truth (John 4:24, *KJV*).

In the beginning was the Word, and the Word was with God, and the Word was God. The same was in the beginning with God. All things were made by him; and without him was not any thing made that was made (John 1:1-3, *KJV*).

2. We did derive our life from this immaterial being. But it came about through a purposeful creative act of God, who made man as a representation of His own likeness (see Gen. 1:26). How could a waveform energy field give rise to highly ordered and complex matter?

3. Sickness, disease and death are a direct result of a disconnection from the source of life—God. However, the disconnection was a result of sin—man's disobedience to his creator—and not because man merely forgot to whom or to what he was connected (see Gen. 3:17-19; Rom. 5:12).

4. The goal of life is to attain oneness with God, but this does not describe oneness in essence. We are not God and we never will be, no matter what level of consciousness we obtain. Instead, we are "at one" with God when our relationship is restored through the atoning work of Christ, and when we yield ourselves fully to Him (see Rom. 3:25).

5. A restored relationship with God does not take place because man reconnects with some sort of universal consciousness within Him. We are not gods who just need enlightenment. Thinking or acting like we are a god is the oldest recorded lie in the Bible. Christianity asserts that there is only one God, and we are separated from Him by sin. Being enlightened would not be enough. We need the Savior who will resolve the enmity that exists between God and mankind.

One Ayurvedic author concluded, "This [Ayurveda] gives rise to a fundamentally different worldview."[35] Indeed it does. The difference between Ayurveda and Christianity is the difference between consciousness and the creator and between union with an energy field and a restored relationship with God through Jesus Christ. Jesus said:

I am come that they might have life, and that they might have it more abundantly (John 10:10, *KJV*).

In place of a joyful reunion with the only true God, Ayurveda and Hinduism offer the counterfeit of a mind completely emptied and a life driven by performance, with the threat of another try for those who don't get it just right this time around.

And this is life eternal, that they might know thee the only true God, and Jesus Christ, whom thou hast sent (John 17:3, *KJV*).

CHAPTER TEN

ALLOPATHY (M.D.)

Allopathic medicine is the predominant medical model in the West. When most people in the United States refer to their medical doctor, they are usually talking about their local allopath. The term *allopathy* was given to medicine around 1800 by Samuel Hahnemann, a German doctor. He named it such because he wanted to draw a clear distinction between his new invention, homeopathy (see chapter 13), and the conventional medicine of his day.[1]

> Allopathy (allo=other): a term applied to that system of therapeutics in which diseases are treated by producing a condition incompatible with or antagonistic to the condition to be cured or alleviated. Also called heteropathy."[2]

EVALUATING THROUGH THE GRID OF HISTORY

Allopathy has had a long and storied history with influences by countless individuals for over 2,500 years. If you were to ask any Western physician to identify the father of modern medicine, he or she would probably say Hippocrates. Born in 460 B.C., this Greek physician had a tremendous impact upon medicine through his emphasis on taking a systematic and thorough history and physical examination. He also is well known for the oath that he penned, variations of which Western physicians have recited ever since.

> I swear by (Greek gods listed) . . . to keep according to my ability and my judgment the following Oath: To consider dear to me as my parents

him who taught me this art; to live in common with him and if necessary to share my goods with him; to look upon his children as my own brothers, to teach them this art if they so desire without fee or written promise; to impart to my sons and the sons of the master who taught me and disciples who have enrolled themselves and have agreed to the rules of the profession, but these alone, the precepts and the instruction. I will prescribe regimen for the good of my patients according to my ability and my judgment and never do harm to anyone. To please no one will I prescribe a deadly drug, nor give advice, which may cause his death. Nor will I give a woman a pessary to procure abortion, but I will preserve the purity of my life and my art. I will not cut for stone, even for patients in whom the disease is manifest; I will leave this operation to be performed by practitioners (specialists in this art). In every house where I come I will enter only for the good of my patients, keeping myself far from all intentional ill-doing and all seduction, and especially from the pleasures of love with women or with men, be they free or slaves. All that may come to my knowledge in the exercise of my profession or outside of my profession in daily commerce with men, which ought not to be spread abroad, I will keep secret and will never reveal. If I keep this oath faithfully, may I enjoy my life and practice my art, respected by all men and in all times; but if I swerve from it or violate it, may the reverse be my lot.[3]

Hippocrates got the philosophy of medicine that he practiced primarily from Pythagoras. In 530 B.C., 70 years before Hippocrates, Pythagoras reacted to Greek theology with its childish gods, quit the medical profession that based its approach upon this pagan system and traveled east looking for truth and a better approach to healing. He came back with beliefs that bear a striking resemblance to Ayurveda and Hinduism.

First, Pythagoras embraced the doctrine of "transmigration of souls," known to us as reincarnation. He also returned convinced that the cosmos was orderly and balanced mathematically, with particular emphasis on the number four. He believed there were four basic elements, four seasons, four qualities and four body humors (fluids). Instead of the three Ayurvedic doshas, he came up with four types of humors by dropping air (vata), adding blood and dividing bile into two types, yellow and black.

It is interesting to note that several hundred years later, Theophrastus, a pupil of Aristotle, connected personalities to these four humors. Those who had blood as their predominant humor were said to be sanguine. Likewise, those with a preponderance of phlegm were referred to as phlegmatic. Black bile was melancholic and yellow bile was choleric. Theophrastus believed that one should treat the personality of the patient, not the disease. This concept of four basic personality types, which has become popular among Western Christians, is traceable back to ancient Ayurvedic thought.

As in Ayurveda, Pythagoras taught that disease developed when one humor was out of balance with the others. Treatment involved eliminating the humor that was in excess. For example, when someone had a fever, they were said to possess a blood excess (referred to as a plethora). This led to the practices of leeches and venesection (opening the veins and allowing them to drain) to reduce this excess evil humor and bring it back into balance with the others.

Hippocrates embraced humoral theory and passed it on to physicians of succeeding generations, the most notable of which was Claudius Galen. Born in A.D. 129, Galen became known as the physician to the emperors. Beginning with Marcus Aurelius, Galen served as the personal physician to five Roman emperors. Not only was Galen's position the envy of the medical world, he also dominated the public scene, conducting animal dissections before large audiences to authenticate humoral theory. He wrote over 400 books, 83 of which survive to this day. Galen died in A.D. 199, and with his death, medicine entered its Dark Ages.

The Dark Ages

We say the Dark Ages because for centuries following Galen, no physician or scientist dared to challenge his thinking; his curriculum vitae was too formidable. Thus, despite its Ayurvedic/Hindu origins, humoral theory along with Galen's faulty interpretations dominated Western medicine for another 1,600 years!

However, with the advent of the Renaissance, the grip of Galen and humoral theory on Western medicine began to weaken slightly as a few brave souls ventured to challenge the status quo. In 1514, Vesalius conducted secret dissections on human cadavers and discovered numerous errors in Galen's dogma. In 1615, William Harvey proclaimed that blood circulated back to the heart, contrary to what Galen had taught. Upon his invention of the microscope in the 1700s, van Leeuwenhoek discovered the invisible world of "animalcules," thereby opening up a whole new realm of understanding the role of germs in the cause of infectious disease. Light was beginning to dawn on the world of medicine.[4]

But despite all of these advances (and many more), humoral theory still dominated Western medicine well into the 1800s. As always, it was associated with extremely harsh measures for removing excess or evil humors:

> Thus, in Germany, doctors indulged in the most audacious and obscure philosophical speculations, even with their fingers on their dying patients' pulse. In England, John . . . Brown's disciples [prescribed] opium by the pound. "Thousands of sick people, and among them some of the most hopeful young persons, fell victim to the opium habit." Italy was dominated by Rasori's system of the *constrastimolo* (counter-excitation): he treated inflammation of the lungs by tapping daily a pound of the patient's blood and then dosing him with 220 grains of digitalis, until finally Nature's resistance was broken and death put an end to the treatment. In France, the bloodletters raged for a long time, until they reached the culmination of their triumph in the butcheries perpetrated by Broussais. On the leech market, deals were made running into millions of these animals. In 1802, a doctor described the activities of the barbers: "Almost every week a wretched barber arrives and lets it be known from house to house that there will be a good bloodletting today; with mendacious powers of persuasion, he cozens the poor out of their groschens, and then they let him deprive them of their most vital excitations. I have known such fellows, who seat their patients in a row, open their veins one after another, and then when all have been opened start bandaging the first: the last of the row sits there with an open vein until all the others have been bandaged. Even some victim's fainting cannot move this cruel monster to depart from his cruel order."[5]

Even George Washington, America's beloved first president, discovered too late the worthlessness of the humoral medicine of his day. Having contracted what was probably a strep infection, his doctors applied a blister to the already inflamed throat and drained so much of his blood that the last of it came "slow and thick." Thus, the "bulletproof George Washington," who had survived countless battles involving numerous attempts on his life, did not recognize that he needed the same divine protection from his own physicians that he had sought and received on the battlefield.[6]

Fortunately, as the nineteenth century progressed and many new discoveries were made, allopathy discarded its humoral theory. However, as we explained in the first chapter of this book, medicine does not exist without a belief system. When humoralism was finally rejected, it was replaced by the religion of science.

EVALUATING THROUGH THE GRID OF FAITH

We don't usually think of science as a religion, but scientists do have a basis for what they believe. In using the term "science," we are not referring to the simple study of nature as described earlier in the book. We are considering the philosophy of science, which we shall refer to as mechanistic science.

Mechanistic science either ignores or denies the existence of God and the reality of the spiritual world. What is real is reserved for only that which exists in the physical realm. Humans are treated only as physical beings, and religion is only good for those who need to believe in some higher power in order to cope with the difficulties of life. Christian doctors would take exception to this of course, but their training would still be limited to natural law with few exceptions. Mechanistic science allies itself closely with evolutionary theory. Some will hang on to their philosophical beliefs even if evidence shows otherwise. Harvard's Nobel prizewinning biologist, George Wald, said:

> There are only two possible explanations as to how life arose: Spontaneous generation arising to evolution or a supernatural creative act of God. . . . There is no other possibility. Spontaneous generation was scientifically disproved 120 years ago by Louis Pasteur and others, but that just leaves us with only one other possibility . . . that life came as a supernatural act of creation by God, but I can't accept that philosophy, because I don't believe in God. Therefore, I choose to believe in that which I know is scientifically impossible, spontaneous generation leading to evolution.[7]

Obviously, to such an individual, science is more than just the study of nature. It has become his religion, or at least the manner in which he practices it and seeks evidence to justify his belief. Since someone's worldview or religious belief system provides the paradigm by which data is interpreted and conclusions are made, it should seem easy to understand how an atheistic evolutionist and a scientist who acknowledges the creator could look at the same data but reach different conclusions.

I (Michael) recall one medical-school professor who criticized the design of the knee joint, saying that it worked well for us when we were on all fours but now that we are upright it is quite unsuitable. That's ridiculous. For one thing, if that were true, our ancestors would have stayed on all fours, since evolutionary theory dictates that a species would not have made such a modification unless it would have made him stronger and more fit to survive. Second, it does not square with reality. Try walking on all fours for awhile. Do your knees feel more comfortable in this position or when you are walking upright as God designed you to walk? My professor was violating his own assertion, even as he stood upright while giving that lecture. His religious views were shaping how he taught science.

Evaluating Through the Wholistic Grid

Summarizing allopathic medicine into one cohesive approach is impossible. Modern Western medicine involves a myriad of approaches, all claiming to be the most scientific or effective. However, a few characteristics are predominant throughout the profession and are useful for us to understand.

1. **Biomedical.** Allopathic medicine is mechanistic. It looks almost exclusively at the physical realm for the cause of disease and for its treatment. In many cases, this is appropriate, since numerous health problems have a purely physical cause. However, sometimes the need to express all of life in purely physical terms borders on the absurd, as noted in a recent *National Public Radio* commentary. The latest diagnosis to come to the broadcaster's attention was "late night eaters syndrome." The broadcaster explained that since he "suffered" from this "condition," he was comforted by the fact that it was finally given an official name by a professional medical

society. However, he also confessed that he felt bad for Satan, since the old devil was receiving progressively less credit for man's vices as medicine was able to label more and more of man's sins with biomedical diagnoses. "For example," he said, "Instead of inattentiveness and lack of self-discipline, patients are now diagnosed with attention deficit disorder. Rather than calling a child's angry, hateful behavior sin, it is more comfortable to classify him as conduct disorder and, if it persists, antisocial." In some cases, a biomedical diagnosis for a problem related to the spirit and soul may be appropriate, such as when kidney failure results in a buildup of toxins to such an extent that thinking is impaired.

2. **Disease focused.** Illness occurs in an individual because a disease has overtaken that person. Therefore, the disease must be opposed. Either it is removed from the body through surgery, or it is opposed with drugs or some other physical agent, such as radiation or laser treatment. Look again at our definition.

> Allopathy (allo=other): a term applied to that system of therapeutics in which diseases are treated by producing a condition incompatible with or antagonistic to the condition to be cured or alleviated. Also called heteropathy.[8]

Allopathic philosophy becomes particularly evident when one looks at the classification of allopathic drugs. Almost all categories begin with the letter "a" for "anti": antibiotics, antifungals, antivirals, antacids, antihypertensives, anti-inflammatory agents, and on and on they go. Disease is the focus and the treatment given is to oppose the disease.

3. **The body does not have the capacity to heal itself.** This may not totally be embraced by every doctor, but functionally that is the operating belief in practice. It has profound implications on how allopathic medicine conducts its treatments and explains the lack of emphasis on wellness and prevention. In recent years, allopaths have embraced the nonallopathic notion that some diseases can be prevented with a prudent lifestyle. However, as soon as a disease does occur, allopaths tend to revert back to their old paradigm, mounting the "white steed"

of modern medicine once again to attack the disease, rather than seeking to understand how to cooperate with the laws of nature in assisting the body's own God-given efforts to heal itself.

EVALUATING THROUGH THE GRID OF SCIENCE

Since the National Library of Medicine catalogs somewhere over 400,000 entries annually, it is impossible for us to examine the scientific basis for every dimension of Western allopathic medicine. Instead, we will summarize its scientific merit in light of the precepts upon which it is based.

> In allopathy, disease is the focus and the treatment given is to oppose the disease.

Just as is true of any other medical philosophy, allopathic medicine works best when its underlying presuppositions match the true underlying cause of the disease in question. Therefore, allopathy is most effective when the condition being addressed is primarily physical in nature and when one or more of the following conditions apply.

1. **Acute crisis.** This is when a life or organ system is threatened, such as with a heart attack, stroke, new onset diabetes, life-threatening infection or trauma. For example, if someone is hit by a car, suffers multiple fractures and is bleeding profusely, they need allopathic treatment. The disease process needs to be opposed quickly and effectively in order to stabilize the patient and to minimize further damage. Bleeding needs to be stopped and fractures need to be realigned so that they can heal. Likewise, if a 55-year-old man develops excruciating chest pain that radiates into his left arm and is accompanied by nausea, vomiting and shortness of breath, he is probably having a heart attack. Despite the fact that most heart attacks are lifestyle related, this is probably not the time to call a nutritionist. What he needs is a good allopathic cardiologist to quickly make the diagnosis and give him a clot-busting drug to remove the blockage in his coronary artery so

that blood flow can once again be restored to his deficient heart muscle. Note: Should he survive and be discharged from the hospital, he should probably seek counsel from others who understand the root causes of heart disease (diet, exercise, spiritual needs, relational issues, fear, etc.), since those considerations are inherently nonallopathic.

I (Michael) recall being paged to the minor-illness ward during residency to evaluate a sick soldier. This young man had developed a fever that would not respond to Tylenol and, therefore, I was called. By the time I arrived on the ward, this otherwise physically fit 20-year-old man was comatose; he would not respond to attempts to awaken him. His temperature had now risen to over 104, and his skin was covered with a fine pinpoint purple rash. Immediately I ordered him down to the intensive care unit where we performed a spinal tap and confirmed our suspicions—meningitis. As quickly as possible, we placed him on high doses of antibiotics to combat the infection. Had we waited a few hours, he would have died.

In such cases in which dramatic, heroic intervention is necessary to spare life or limb, allopathy shines. Indeed, those are the situations that line up most closely with its paradigm.

2. **Congenital disease in which surgical correction is possible.** Not long ago, a good friend of ours gave birth to what at first appeared to be a healthy young boy. However, before long, it became evident that something was wrong. A trip to his doctor revealed a congenital heart defect in which his aorta and pulmonary arteries were improperly developed. Fifteen years ago, I watched children die after their heart surgeries failed to correct the same diagnosis. But with major advances in pediatric heart surgery, this boy's problem was—from indications nearly two years later—completely corrected surgically.

3. **Advanced disease.** With some cancers, we know that the underlying causes include diet and other lifestyle issues such as stress. Despite this, when someone is diagnosed with cancer, it often needs to be treated allopathically. While there are a few exceptions to this rule, surgery tends to be the most effective allopathic approach. In general,

if surgery cannot completely remove the cancer, the prognosis with allopathic treatment (or any other treatment for that matter) is usually poor.

This statement regarding poor prognoses is made with the knowledge that there are claims of cures for cancer being made by some in alternative medicine. I (Michael) have personally toured a number of these alternative treatment centers in the U.S. and Mexico and interviewed their directors. While some patients are legitimately healed of their cancer at these facilities, I came away with the conclusion that there is no surefire "miracle cure" for this dreaded disease. However, in all fairness to these alternative treatment centers, they usually get patients who have tried conventional allopathic medicine without success, so they seek alternative medicine in the late stages of illness. It would be a good research project to randomly select cancer patients at the onset of their disease: One group would try alternative diet and exercise programs that included spiritual interventions in their lifestyle and relationship with God, while the other group tried allopathic medicine.

> Maintaining the position that virtually all disease has a physical cause essentially renders God and the patient's faith irrelevant to their condition.

4. **Replacement therapy.** In some cases, Western medicine does not really practice allopathically, particularly when it properly identifies the original design and seeks to work in harmony with it. For example, such is the case with insulin replacement therapy. Although the underlying cause for juvenile onset diabetes has not been identified, the result of this disease is the inability of the pancreas to produce its own insulin. When scientific research properly isolated the missing hormone and discovered how to produce an exact copy, it was seeking to work with God's design. To the degree that this is possible, the treatment will be effective.

5. **Relief of symptoms.** Allopathic medicine is often criticized for treating only symptoms. Sometimes this is needed. For example, I

(Michael) used to suffer miserably with hay fever until I discovered several underlying factors that contributed to my illness. Once these were addressed, my hay fever completely disappeared. However, about once or twice a year, my symptoms tend to come back for a brief time, particularly when I have violated those things that I know contribute to my disease. But I know that even if I correct those violations, it will take some time for them to have their effect. When I have an allergy attack, I want immediate relief. Therefore, allopathic medicine is best at offering me that near-instant relief, even if it is temporary and does not truly cure my problem.

While allopathic medicine tends to do well under the above conditions, it does not when it ventures outside of them. This is especially true when it comes to prevention, degenerative disorders and those involving the spirit and soul. Furthermore, allopathic medicine has a tremendous overreliance upon medications. Except as replacement therapy, drugs do not tend to correct the underlying condition. In addition, adverse drug reactions have been estimated to be the fourth leading cause of death in hospitalized patients.[9]

EVALUATING THROUGH THE GRID OF SPIRITUAL DISCERNMENT

It goes without saying that there is a great need in allopathic medicine to acknowledge the spiritual dimension. Maintaining the position that virtually all disease has a physical cause essentially renders God and the patient's faith irrelevant to their condition—a proposition that is not only unwise from a spiritual standpoint but also may result in a very misled medical approach.

While it appears that a shift is taking place, it is mostly due to recognition of the mind-body connection, which represents a transition toward Eastern thought rather than toward a biblical paradigm. We consider this alternative to be even more dangerous spiritually than the former ignorance. It is probably spiritually safer to utilize an allopath who deals strictly in the biomedical model than to employ the services of one who is looking to an Eastern paradigm to explain what occurs beyond the physical.

CONCLUSION

Allopathy is the scientific orthodox medicine of the West. When compared to other medical systems, we believe it (along with osteopathy) to be the best system in the world today, particularly in the treatment of conditions that line up most closely with its paradigm. However, it is not Christian medicine, particularly when one considers its infatuation with a purely mechanistic model of man and its rejection of a biblical worldview. It has its limitations and, as we will see in some cases, is better spurned for a more effective approach.

CHAPTER ELEVEN

OSTEOPATHY (D.O.)

*As I have spent thirty years of my life reading and following rules and
remedies used for curing, and learned in sorrow it was useless to listen
to their claims, for instead of getting good, I obtained much harm
therefrom, I asked for, and obtained a mental divorce from them,
and I want it to be understood that drugs and I are as far apart as the
East is from the West; now, and forever. Henceforth I will follow
the dictates of nature in all I say and write.*

A.T. STILL, 1899

EVALUATING THROUGH THE GRID OF HISTORY

Osteopathy was founded in 1874 by Andrew Taylor Still, M.D. A.T. was born in
1828 in Lee County, Virginia, to a circuit-riding preacher and physician. He
eventually apprenticed in medicine under his father. But while serving in the
Civil War as a field surgeon, he witnessed the ineffectiveness of medicine
against infectious disease and began to question his allopathic training. His dis-
enchantment peaked in 1864 when he lost all three of his children to an epidemic of meningitis. (His first wife had already died at a young age in 1859.)

Instead of quitting medicine, he went back to studying anatomy and physiology, both by textbook and through cadaver dissection. During the next 10
years, he developed several new concepts particularly involving the importance
of spinal alignment and its proper circulation. Eventually, in 1874, he publicly
announced his discoveries, giving his new medical approach the name of

osteopathy. In 1892, with the assistance of an M.D., Still obtained a charter from the state of Missouri and opened a medical school in Kirksville. In order to draw a distinction between his graduates and those with allopathic training, he called them osteopaths and gave them the degree of D.O. (doctor of osteopathy).

During a time when allopathic medicine was still notoriously ineffective—when it was just learning concepts of antisepsis and prior to the advent of the antibiotic era—the popularity of osteopathy exploded. Soon there were schools all over the country. However, quality control was poor, so many closed down (a problem in many allopathic schools at that time as well). Yet the profession survived and continued to grow stronger despite significant antagonism from its allopathic brethren. Today osteopaths hold unrestricted licenses to practice medicine in all 50 states. While many of its graduates enter the primary-care fields of medicine, osteopaths represent every subspecialty known.

EVALUATING THROUGH THE GRID OF FAITH

The son of a circuit-riding preacher, A.T. Still came from a strong Christian background and was probably a believer himself. In his *Philosophy of Osteopathy*, he repeatedly refers to the God of the Bible and writes, "I will use the word that the theologian often uses when asked whom Christ died for, the answer universally is, ALL."[1]

While osteopathic concepts find good compatibility with Scripture, like their M.D. counterparts, the majority of D.O.'s do not identify themselves as Christians. Therefore, the underlying worldview of many osteopaths tends to be similar to that of many allopaths—mechanistic science.

EVALUATING THROUGH THE WHOLISTIC GRID

Osteopathy does not have the same philosophical roots that allopathic medicine does.

Osteopathy: a system of therapy founded by Andrew Taylor Still (1828-1917) and based on the theory that the body is capable of making its own remedies against disease and other toxic conditions when it is in normal structural relationship and has favorable environmental conditions and adequate nutrition. It utilizes generally accepted physical, medicinal and surgical methods of diagnosis and therapy, while placing chief emphasis on the importance of normal body mechanics and manipulative methods of detecting and correcting faulty structure.[2]

Doctor Still articulated several fundamental concepts that underlie osteopathic medicine.

1. The human body was designed by a wise creator. Note: this concept is not generally stated by secular writers articulating foundational principles of osteopathy. However, it is clearly implied and repeatedly affirmed by osteopathy's founder.

   I love God because His works are perfect and trustworthy . . . I am convinced that God has done His work completely.[3]

2. The body has the inherent capacity to heal itself. This is in stark contrast to allopathic philosophy and is why many osteopaths are more open to concepts in nutrition than their allopathic brethren. Occasionally, an allopath, such as Dr. Richard C. Cabot of Harvard, would agree with Still.

God and the wisdom of the human body constitute 90 percent of the hope of patients to recover. The body simply has a superwisdom which is biased in favor of life rather than death. . . . These are the powers on which all of us depend for life. . . . I earnestly recommend to the medical profession to let the patient know of this great force that is working within him.[4]

3. The body is a unit, a complete whole. When one part is impaired, all parts are affected.
4. Structure and function are related. When there is an abnormality in structure (such as the bony skeleton), this will impair the body's function in some way.
5. Osteopathic manipulation is used to restore normal structure and, thereby, function. Dr. Still independently discovered and introduced

concepts of spinal manipulation to America (D. D. Palmer and chiropractic came 21 years later; see chapter 12).

For example, in patients with asthma, an osteopath may examine the area of the spine between the shoulder blades to look for dysfunction. The reason for this is that the sympathetic nervous-system chain that controls the airway smooth muscle is located in this region. In some cases, by correcting dysfunction of the spine, performance of the sympathetic nervous system can be improved. This in turn can lead to a reduction in smooth muscle spasm and, therefore, improves the symptoms of asthma.

The osteopath first seeks physiological perfection of form, by normally adjusting the osseous frame work, so that all arteries may deliver blood to nourish and construct all parts. Also that the veins may carry away all impurities dependent upon them for renovation. Also that the nerves of all classes may be free and unobstructed while applying the powers of life and motion to all divisions.[5]

> For those doctors who consistently practice with osteopathic philosophy, spinal manipulation tends to be employed as a significant part of their practice.

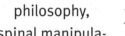

In addition to the above is craniosacral therapy, a dimension of osteopathic therapy that was developed by William Sutherland, D.O., in the early 1900s. Sutherland believed that the bones of the skull (cranium) were not fused at adulthood but moved very, very slightly in an automatic rhythmic pattern, much like our lungs breathe in and out. He believed that this motion was linked with the movement of cerebrospinal fluid (CSF) and that impaired cranial motion (typically occurring as a result of trauma) could result in headaches, sinus trouble, recurrent ear infections or a host of other problems in the body. Craniosacral therapy is practiced by a small subset of osteopaths and other healing professions such as chiropractic, which has also adopted its concepts.

Despite the fact that these principles are at the foundation of osteopathic medicine, most osteopathic training today is a carbon copy of that which is provided in allopathic schools. Purely osteopathic concepts are largely confined to one specific series of courses on manipulative medicine during the medical school years (and occasional osteopathic educational programs after graduation). Many osteopaths are trained by allopaths and vice versa. For example, my (Michael's) family practice residency included M.D.'s and D.O.'s among its faculty, and my board certification is with the American Board of Family Practice, an allopathic organization. Therefore, for the most part, the majority of what we have written in regard to allopathic medicine applies to osteopathic medicine as well.

For those D.O.'s who consistently practice with osteopathic philosophy, spinal manipulation tends to be employed as a significant part of their practice. These osteopaths are usually in primary care and many participate in associations that emphasize spinal manipulation, such as the American Association of Osteopathy (AAO).

EVALUATING THROUGH THE GRID OF SCIENCE

Once again, most of what was written in regard to allopathy applies to osteopathy. However, depending upon the practitioner, there are differences, since classical osteopathy differs greatly from allopathic medicine. Most significantly, there are numerous studies evaluating the validity of spinal manipulation. Scientific evidence is strong that manipulation is beneficial and effective in the treatment of especially acute pain syndromes of the neck, upper back and lower back and related problems such as headache and lumbar disc.[6]

Data regarding the use of spinal manipulation to treat other diseases, such as asthma,[7] is much less impressive and confined primarily to the osteopathic (and chiropractic) literature. Controlled trials have found that osteopathic manipulation hastened recovery after knee and hip surgery[8] and was more effective than light-touch therapy in shortening the duration of antibiotic use and hospital stay.[9] However, we were able to find virtually no other clinical trials that proved the effectiveness of craniosacral therapy,[10] and more than one indicated that practitioners of this art disagreed with one another when it came to assessing their patients for the craniosacral rhythm.[11]

EVALUATING THROUGH THE GRID OF SPIRITUAL DISCERNMENT

For reasons mentioned in chapter 10, osteopaths tend to share a spiritual profile similar to that of M.D.'s. However, due to their more wholistic philosophy and greater openness to alternative approaches, there may be a greater emphasis on the spiritual dimension in an osteopathic practice. This appears to be particularly true in craniosacral therapy, since some practitioners have postulated that the craniosacral rhythm—that is being felt and manipulated—is the body's vital force or energy field. Therefore, they claim that using New Age "centering" techniques enhances the practice of this art.[12] I (Michael) am personally familiar with a dedicated Christian craniosacral osteopath who resigned his executive position with a leading craniosacral organization because of the insistence of some of its members on teaching centering techniques and in conducting overt New Age activities at their conferences. Once again, vigilance is in order since much of the spiritual influence coming into both allopathic medicine and osteopathic medicine has its roots in Eastern mysticism.

CHAPTER TWELVE

CHIROPRACTIC (D.C.) AND NATUROPATHY (N.D.)

CHIROPRACTIC MEDICINE

Evaluating Through the Grid of History

Chiropractic medicine was invented in 1895 by Daniel David Palmer. Born in the Toronto area in 1845, he moved with his family to Davenport, Iowa, at a young age. Early on, he raised bees and ran a grocery store. Eventually he heard of and became interested in osteopathy (see chapter 11) and began to dabble in various medical philosophies.[1] In the 1880s, he employed himself as a magnetic healer for nine years prior to developing his interest in chiropractic (see chapter 7 and 19 for more information on magnetic healing).[2]

In 1875, he met Dr. Jim Atkinson, who spoke with him about spinal manipulation. However, it wasn't until 21 years later that Palmer actually delved further into the subject. The opportunity presented itself in the form of Harvey Lillard, a deaf janitor who worked in the building where Palmer had an office. Deaf for 17 years, Lillard allowed Palmer to talk him into an examination, particularly after Lillard explained that his deafness had immediately followed a back injury. Upon the examination, Palmer discovered what appeared to be a vertebra that was not in line with the rest. Using his hand, Palmer forced the spinous process of this vertebra back in line with the others. Upon doing so, Lillard's hearing returned.

A short time later, Palmer discovered a displaced vertebra in a patient with heart trouble. With two very different diseases both traced to a problem with spinal alignment, Palmer reasoned that all disease was secondary to this malady and its resultant impingement upon nerves.

He commissioned a local minister to come up with a Greek name for his new invention. Two Greek words were selected, one meaning "hand" and the other meaning "practice," to form the word "chiropractic." Soon thereafter, he founded the Palmer College of Chiropractic Medicine in Davenport. It didn't take long before Palmer experienced intense opposition. Some of it came from within his own ranks, even from his own son Bartlett Joshua (BJ), who conducted a civil war against his father.[3]

Most of the antagonism came from the allopathic profession, however, which had by that time organized into the American Medical Association. Opposition by the American Medical Association (AMA) toward chiropractors was even more intense than what the osteopaths experienced, perhaps because Palmer was not a trained physician. It also may have been due in part to BJ's verbal abuse of the medical profession. He would say that "M.D." stood for "more dope" and "D.C." meant "disease conquered."[4] The AMA banned its members from cooperating professionally with chiropractors. This meant that AMA members were not allowed to refer patients to chiropractors nor were they allowed to cooperate with chiropractors in the care of their patients. This was referred to as the "consultation clause," but was not a policy uniquely directed at chiropractors. Osteopaths and homeopaths experienced the same treatment until the latter half of the twentieth century. On occasion, this policy was carried to absurd lengths, such as when an M.D. was expelled from his local medical society for consulting with his wife because she was a homeopath.[5]

Throughout their history, chiropractors have not sought nor have they obtained full, unrestricted medical licensure (which allows its holder the right to prescribe medicine and do surgery). This has contributed to their remaining outside the mainstream of medicine, which includes hospitals, medical societies and insurance reimbursement. However, that seems to be changing. While there are numerous factors and events that have worked to bring that change about, we will mention two of the most salient.

The first has to do with the actions of the AMA toward the chiropractic profession. In 1990, in *Wilk v. AMA,* the United States Supreme Court affirmed a lower-court ruling that found the AMA guilty of conspiracy to "contain and eliminate" the chiropractic profession. The AMA was required to pay reparations and reverse its ban on interprofessional cooperation between their members and chiropractors.[6]

Another landmark event was the release in 1994 of the *Guidelines for Acute Lower-Back Pain* by the United States Department of Health and Human Services. In this document, a panel of 21 medical doctors and 2 chiropractors concluded that spinal manipulation was effective in the treatment of acute lower-back pain. They recommended that it be either used in combination with or in place of medication for this condition. Furthermore, it found the allopathic treatments of bed rest and traction to be ineffective and cautioned against the use of surgery except in severe cases.[7]

In the intervening years since, chiropractors have been increasingly integrated into the health-care community. Because of their orientation toward the musculoskeletal system, a number have served as physicians for sports teams. Several have joined group practices with M.D.'s, and some have been granted hospital privileges. An increasing number of insurance companies are reimbursing for services provided by chiropractors, particularly with regard to neck and back problems. While chiropractors will probably never have the unrestricted licenses of their osteopathic and allopathic counterparts, the vast majority of them have no desire to go in that direction, which would require a major shift in chiropractic-school curriculum.

Evaluating Through the Grid of Faith

Palmer described his mother as "superstitious as an egg is full of meat."[8] Perhaps that is what influenced him to enter into magnetic healing, which he practiced "for nine years previous to discovering the principles which comprise the method known as chiropractic."[9] Palmer carried these beliefs into chiropractic theory and spoke of the "innate" as a healing force. To what degree he ascribed a spiritual dimension to the innate is not clear, although some who have followed him consider it entirely as such.

Evaluating Through the Wholistic Grid

Chiropractic medicine according to *Dorland's Medical Dictionary* is:

> Chiropractic. Gr. *chiro* = hand; *practic* = to do, practice. A system of therapeutics based upon the claim that disease is caused by an abnormal

function of the nervous system. It attempts to restore normal function of the nervous system by manipulation and treatment of the structures of the human body, especially those of the spinal column.[10]

While A.T. Still emphasized the role of the artery, Palmer focused on the importance of healthy nerve transmission. He believed that all disease was due to an impingement of nerves by misaligned vertebrae.

Displacement of any part of the skeletal frame may press against nerves, which are the channels of communication, intensifying or decreasing their carrying capacity, creating either too much or not enough functioning, an aberration known as disease.[11]

Thus, he articulated the one-cause-one-cure concept that characterized chiropractic medicine throughout most of its history. Restated, it expresses the belief that "the vertebral subluxation (spinal misalignment causing abnormal nerve transmission) is the cause of virtually all disease, and that the chiropractic adjustment (a manual manipulation of the subluxated vertebrae) is its cure."[12]

 Principles of chiropractic medicine are almost identical to the osteopathic concepts from which they are believed to have originated.

Palmer always looked for one specific segment that was misaligned, claiming that this is what made chiropractic superior to osteopathy. More recently, chiropractic has adopted what it refers to as "motion theory," a concept that looks quite osteopathic in that it acknowledges that subluxation always involves more than one single segment and whose significance is found in the dysfunctional motion between these segments.[13]

Chiropractors employ several different methods for adjustment of the spine. But by far the most common utilizes direct thrust, and is known as high velocity low amplitude (HVLA), the same term used by osteopaths. Another concept borrowed from osteopathic research is that of the facilitated segment, which describes how a restricted vertebrae impairs the function of the nearby autonomic nervous-system chain. This concept provides a theoretical basis for how spinal misalignment for motion problems can contribute to disease of other organs (see chapter 11 on osteopathy).[14]

Principles of chiropractic medicine are summarized as follows (most are almost identical to the osteopathic concepts from which they are believed to have originated):

1. Structure and function exist in intimate relation with one another.
2. Structural distortions can cause functional abnormalities.
3. The vertebral subluxation is a significant form of structural distortion and leads to a variety of functional abnormalities.
4. The nervous system plays a prominent role in the restoration and maintenance of proper bodily function.
5. Subluxation influences bodily function primarily through neurologic means.
6. Chiropractic adjustment is a specific and definitive method for the correction of vertebral subluxation.[15]

In addition, chiropractic affirms the innate healing potential of the body, the potential for interference with this natural healing process by the use of drugs and the value of regular exercise and a balanced, natural diet.

Evaluating Through the Grid of Science

There is incontrovertible evidence that spinal manipulation is at least as effective as, if not superior to, allopathic treatment of back and neck pain.[16] Perhaps the most impressive study came out of Canada in a 1985 first-of-its-kind project between J. R. Cassidy, a chiropractor, and W. H. Kirkaldy-Willis, a highly regarded orthopedic surgeon. The study involved nearly 300 subjects who had been totally disabled by back pain for an average of seven years. After daily chiropractic treatment for several weeks, over 70 percent were able to return to work with no restrictions.[17] This is astounding, particularly considering the fact that the vast majority of injured employees who are unable to work for more than one year never return from disability.

Questions still remain in regard to the shared osteopathic and chiropractic concept that spinal dysfunction can contribute in significant ways to the disease of internal organs. A number of studies have been conducted on a small scale, and others are in progress. Overall, the general consensus from controlled trials is that spinal manipulation is of very little benefit for other than musculoskeletal conditions, although, there are case reports that claim otherwise.[18]

While chiropractic manipulation has earned a legitimate degree of respect, the profession often undermines itself with the common practice of combining chiropractic with other approaches, such as applied kinesiology, which do not enjoy the same degree of scientific acceptance. Another common practice is the utilization of passive therapy such as electrical stimulation and ultrasound. While patients appreciate the comfort of these additions to the treatment regimen, there is little evidence to indicate that they actually increase the effectiveness of manipulative therapy. Instead, they probably represent an unnecessary expense to patients and insurance companies.

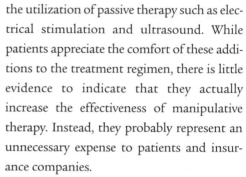

A chiropractor who practices pure chiropractic musculoskeletal medicine— focusing on adjustment of the spine—is operating purely in the physical realm.

Another common unnecessary expense is X rays. Most chiropractors own their own X ray machines and tend to utilize them far more than their osteopathic counterparts. The information that is gleaned from X rays taken purely to assess alignment can usually be obtained through palpation (feeling with the hands) of the spine, something which both osteopaths and chiropractors have been trained to do. X rays taken of the back in the wake of acute strains are almost always normal. Professional organizations and government agencies (such as the American Committee for Health and Policy Research, ACHPR) generally consider back X rays (as well as CT and MRI scans) unnecessary in most cases of acute back pain.[19]

Evaluating Through the Grid of Spiritual Discernment

A chiropractor who practices pure chiropractic musculoskeletal medicine— focusing on adjustment of the spine—is operating purely in the physical realm. However, perhaps because chiropractic has historically been outside of the medical mainstream, and perhaps because many alternative medicine systems (iridology, reflexology, TCM, etc.) do not require a medical license for their practice, there appears to be a greater tendency for chiropractors to get involved in unlicensed approaches that are either mystical, scientifically questionable or both.

NATUROPATHIC MEDICINE

Having spent most of my (Michael's) growing-up years on the West Coast, I arranged several clinical rotations there during the latter part of my medical-school years. However, upon my return to my home state of Washington, I developed severe hay fever (allergic rhinitis). Although I thought my symptoms would improve after I left the area, they only seemed to get worse no matter where I lived. My hay fever got so bad that I required antihistamines on a daily basis in order to get some relief from the symptoms. Since these drugs made me very drowsy, I tried to use them as little as possible, relying instead on nasal steroid sprays.

Several years later, while attending a Christian medical conference in 1989, I met a midwife who was successfully employing nutrition for a number of common clinical problems. Since I had had an interest in nutrition for a number of years but had not received training during my formal medical education on how to integrate nutrition with the practice of medicine, I questioned her extensively and began educating myself.

The first book I read was *The Yeast Syndrome* by Drs. Trowbridge and Walker (Bantam Books, 1986). I learned about the common problem of intestinal yeast infections. While the authors seemed to attribute almost every imaginable chronic problem to this underlying malady, I was somewhat intrigued, since allergies made the list. Furthermore, it seemed logical that yeast could be my problem because the hay fever often followed the use of antibiotics. Due to an underlying internal birth defect that was not corrected until I was 11 years old, I had been on antibiotics almost every day of my life until my surgery at age 11. Looking back, I also recalled that my hay fever symptoms had developed shortly after taking a course of antibiotics.

While most authors on the yeast problem claim that there is no reliable lab test to diagnose intestinal yeast overgrowth, I found a couple of research articles that indicated otherwise. I located Diagnos-Techs—a clinical laboratory in the Seattle area that specializes in this sort of testing—and provided the stool culture that confirmed my suspicions. Upon undergoing a treatment regimen to eliminate the yeast, my hay fever symptoms dramatically improved.

As I explored further in both lay and research publications, I discovered other factors that can contribute to hay fever, including stress, food allergies and deficiencies in antioxidants. As these problems were identified and corrected, my hay fever completely resolved. Occasionally, particularly when I fail to get adequate rest or maintain at least the semblance of a prudent diet, my symptoms may briefly return. When they do, I know the lifestyle issues that have contributed to the hay fever symptoms.

My problem with hay fever has been a good motivator toward prudent behavior. Furthermore, it has opened my eyes to the value of other health-care approaches. Allopathic and osteopathic medicine were ineffective in addressing the underlying root causes to my allergy problems. The most effective approach I found for addressing allergic rhinitis was outside the mainstream of these two systems. Even though I never consulted a naturopathic doctor, it was their paradigm in which I found answers. One case study, however, does not constitute good scientific research, and that is true for any other personal testimony we give.

Evaluating Through the Grid of History

The founder of naturopathic medicine in the United States was Benedict Lust, a young German who immigrated here in 1892 (the same year A.T. Still opened the first osteopathic medical school in Kirksville, Missouri). As a teenager, Benedict became seriously ill with tuberculosis and was sent to Sebastian Kneipp, a renowned Austrian priest and hydrotherapist, who successfully treated Lust for his disease using water treatments (hot and cold water, saunas, sitz baths, colonics, etc.). Impressed with Father Kneipp's natural approach, Lust came to the U.S. at age 23 with the purpose of bringing Kneipp's hydrotherapy to the States.[20]

Lust was not the first to advocate natural-healing methods west of the Atlantic. By the time he arrived in the U.S., several significant movements were well under way.

- Sylvester Graham had been preaching messages on temperance and hygiene, emphasizing a vegetarian diet, whole grains and a moderate lifestyle.
- Russell Trall, M.D., had taken up the hygienic cause and founded a school in 1852 to train physicians in this healing art. During this

time, the concept of a healthy immune system to protect oneself
from infectious disease became incorporated into the natural health
movement.

- John Tilden, M.D., proposed the idea of "autointoxication," referring
  to the detrimental effect of fecal matter remaining too long in the
  digestive tract. Tilden suggested excess constipation would cause tox-
  emia, and he blamed meat as the greatest contributor.

- The nature cure movement emphasized natural living, a vegetarian
  diet and the use of light and air. This latter approach became popular in the late 1800s and early 1900s through the influence of Henry
  Lindlahr, a Chicago businessman-turned-physician.

In 1896, four years after his arrival in the United States, Lust matriculated
at Universal Osteopathic College of New York, eventually graduating and
obtaining a license as a D.O. In addition to his osteopathic training, he also
schooled in chiropractic. He opened the first health-food store in the country.
In 1902, he named his natural approach naturopathy and founded its first
school. At the American School of Naturopathy, he integrated a variety of
noninvasive healing concepts and disciplines noted above. To these were eventually added homeopathy, herbal medicine and Christian Science.

Until his death in 1945, Lust aggressively promoted the natural-healing
concepts embodied in naturopathy.[21] For a season, his fledgling medical discipline flourished, with conventions in the 1920s boasting as many as 10,000
practitioners. However, with the death of Lust and the tremendous growth in
the pharmaceutical industry and in allopathic medicine after World War II,
naturopathy all but disappeared until natural-healing methods experienced a
resurgence once again in the 1970s.

Evaluating Through the Grid of Faith

With naturopathy, there is no single religious system underlying its philosophy
other than perhaps eclecticism. Eclectics claim allegiance to no particular faith
or medical dogma. Instead, in the same way that they consider various approaches to medicine, they tend to sample cafeteria-style from a variety of beliefs
according to their liking.

With regard to personal beliefs, there is great variation between naturopathic practitioners. Some Christian naturopaths find good consistency

between natural-healing concepts and a biblical paradigm (natural law, personal responsibility, lifestyle issues, treating the whole person, the physician as counselor, etc.). However, based upon the practices they employ, a majority of N.D.'s appear to either be eclectic or Eastern in their religious beliefs.

Evaluating Through the Wholistic Grid

Benedict Lust was an effective leader and entrepreneur. However, most of the ideas embodied in naturopathy were not his own. Indeed, naturopaths trace their history at least as far back as Hippocrates, who was the first to use the term *vis medicatrix naturae*, which means "the healing power of nature." While there are certainly some approaches employed by naturopaths that are consistent with this concept of the body's self-healing capacity, in reality, naturopaths tend to be receptive to anything that is noninvasive (i.e., that employs something other than drugs or surgery), even if the philosophical system upon which it is based has very little to do with true natural healing.

Several key principles underlie naturopathic philosophy.

1. The vast majority of illness is due to an accumulation of toxins.
2. Look for the cause, especially in the violation of the laws of nature (diet, habits, etc.).

Naturopaths tend to focus more on evaluating the health of the body's basic organ systems and using laboratory testing to assess how well these systems are functioning.

To that end, naturopaths tend to be less concerned than allopaths with giving the patient's disease a name (i.e., diagnosis). Instead, they tend to focus more on evaluating the health of the body's basic organ systems (such as the digestive system, the detoxification functions of the liver and kidneys, hormonal balance, the stress system, etc.) and using laboratory testing to assess how well these systems are functioning. For example, in my own experience with allergies, I (Michael) did not focus on the diagnosis of hay fever but rather looked for underlying system problems that, if impaired, could contribute to a poorly functioning immune system, which resulted in the hay fever symptoms.

In general, naturopaths tend to believe that standard allopathic laboratory testing is limited in its value at promoting optimum health because it is either too insensitive or it does not measure factors that reflect proper function of certain body systems, especially those involved with toxin removal, the immune system or digestion. Naturopaths tend to look much closer at bowel function to assess for poor digestion (which may be caused by inadequate stomach acid or digestive enzymes) or overgrowth of pathogens (disease-causing organisms such as bacteria, parasites or yeasts, as described in my own experience).

3. Treat the whole person in their mental, emotional, spiritual and physical environments. (In reality, the physical tends to get the preponderance of attention. How the spirit and soul issues are addressed (if at all) varies tremendously among naturopaths and depends upon the individual practitioner's belief system.)
4. The body has the inherent capacity to heal itself. Some naturopaths attribute this more to a mystical vital-force principle rather than to a law of nature.
5. Do no harm. Naturopaths emphasize wellness, prevention and non-invasive treatment.
6. The doctor functions as a teacher and counselor; patients are responsible for their own health.

Therapeutic approaches are "Virtually any therapy that is consistent with these guiding principles (is used). . . . In other words, the naturopathic physician uses therapies that support the body's inherent healing processes."[22] The following 11 approaches are examples of what a naturopath might practice:

1. **Diet.** A natural, unrefined diet emphasizing organically grown foods intake with limited or no meat intake. Naturopaths tend to advocate vegetarianism (see chapter 17).
2. **Exercise.** (See chapter 17.)
3. **Rest.** As in the forms of regular sleep, relaxation and meditation (see chapters 7 and 20).
4. **Detoxification.** This may include fasting and/or cleansing of the bowel and body with herbs, enemas, etc. When someone is eating,

they are said to be in an *anabolic* mode. In other words, they are building up the body and its stores of nutrients and energy. In fasting (drinking only water), an individual is in a *catabolic* mode. They are breaking things down and using up their body's stores of nutrients and energy, which is also thought by naturopaths to be necessary to cleanse the body of toxins deposited in stored fat. Fasting from a few days to several weeks has been a mainstay of the natural-hygiene movement since the mid-1800s. I (Michael) watched this process firsthand with my own mother. Suffering from high blood pressure, atrial fibrillation (an irregularity of the heart) and a tendency to produce blood clots, my mother was on four medications and still unable to control those conditions. She underwent a several-week fast under the watchful eye of David Scott, a Cleveland chiropractor and naturopath, who had been monitoring therapeutic fasts on patients for several decades. Two years later, she is off all of her medications and none of her three diseases have returned.

5. **Plant-based remedies.** Herbs and botanicals are two popular remedies (see chapter 18).

6. **Homeopathy.** (Addressed in chapter 13.)

7. **Hydrotherapy.** Simply stated, hydrotherapy is the therapeutic use of water in any form. In chapter 8, I (Michael) shared the story of my pastor, Larry Cornett, and how the Lord used an injection procedure (prolotherapy) to spare him from neck surgery. Several years later, Pastor Cornett reinjured his neck and required prolotherapy once again. However, unlike the first time, he did not improve, even after a series of three treatments. I was becoming concerned that he would require surgery after all. Then one Saturday I received an unexpected phone call from his mother who suggested that I have Larry take hot water therapy. Lois explained to me that she had recently struggled with a shoulder problem and found that the water had really helped her condition. Despite the fact that I had never felt the need to prescribe this sort of therapy to a neck-injection patient, her idea made sense to me, as I recalled that Pastor Cornett had not been able to move his neck much at all due to the severity of his pain. Recognizing that motion was necessary in order for his treatment to work and for him to heal, I had him get into a hot tub with water up to his chin.

I encouraged him to spend at least 30 minutes a day in the water and to gently move his arms and neck around, something which the hot water enabled him to finally do. He took his first treatment on Monday, and his pain was significantly less almost immediately. He had more motion in his neck and, for the first time in three months, he was able to get a good night's sleep. By Sunday, he was back in the pulpit again with no further need of injections, pain medication or other therapy. In this case, the hot water was all that was needed to complete his treatment puzzle.

8. **Acupuncture.** (See chapter 14.)
9. **Physical modalities.** Treatments using heat, cold, sunlight, electricity, etc. Let's consider the use of heat. The body's normal response to infection is to raise its temperature. This helps fight the infection in at least two ways. First, some bacteria and viruses are unable to survive at higher temperatures. Second, the body's immune system functions with greater effectiveness at Fahrenheit temperatures between 101-103 degrees.[23]

   Therefore, naturopaths try to mimic these conditions as a mode of therapy. I (Michael) saw this while touring clinics in Mexico. Patients enclosed themselves up to their necks in personal "hot boxes" that raised their body temperature to feverlike states. Whole-body heat is not only being used to fight infection but other diseases as well, such as cancer. In the early 1900s, orthopedic surgeon William Colles, M.D., noticed that tumors shrank in patients who developed fevers while awaiting surgery to remove their cancer. He did some experimenting, eventually isolating substances from two different bacteria that triggered fevers in patients infected by them. These eventually became known as Colles' toxins and are still used today by some alternative clinics to induce hyperthermia in cancer patients.[24] Some allopathic cancer centers are now conducting experiments in the use of hyperthermia as well.

10. **Massage.** (See chapter 19.)
11. **Spinal manipulation.** (See chapters 11 and 12.)

Therapeutically, N.D.'s use virtually every known natural therapy: diet, therapeutic nutrition, botanical medicine (primarily European, Native

American and Chinese), physical therapy, spinal manipulation, lifestyle counseling, exercise therapy, homeopathy, acupuncture, psychological and family counseling, and hydrotherapy.[25]

Evaluating Through the Grid of Science

There is very little research in regard to how successful naturopathy is as a profession at treating disease. This would be difficult to do, since there is not one consistent approach to treatment. In order to assess its effectiveness, one needs to look at each individual treatment or diagnostic approach. Diet and exercise, meditation and relaxation, herbal medicine, homeopathy, acupuncture, massage and spinal manipulation are addressed later in this book. What are left are hydrotherapy, physical modalities and detoxification.

Hydrotherapy. In many ways, hydrotherapy is a major treatment modality for many medical systems, not just naturopathy. Ice is used to reduce swelling after an injury. Hot compresses increase circulation. Whirlpools help increase the mobility of stiff joints. Sitz baths are commonly employed for the treatment of hemorrhoids or to soothe and stimulate healing after an episiotomy. Doctors often encourage drinking plenty of water to improve general health or to aid in the treatment of specific conditions, such as bladder infections and kidney stones.

Water is essential to life and also to the practice of medicine. Naturopaths like Benjamin Lust have always appreciated its value, although they have tended to make grander claims as to the healing potential of water than other medical systems were ready to acknowledge. One note of caution regarding hydrotherapy—be careful regarding the risk of infection from tubs and whirlpools. During a literature search for articles on hydrotherapy and disease, there were very few citations other than reports of outbreaks of bacterial infection.

Physical Modalities (Heat, Cold, Sun, Electricity). Saunas have played a significant role in Scandinavian cultures for centuries (perhaps because they are so far north, they're looking for a warm place to sit awhile). Having Scandinavian backgrounds ourselves, we can attest to the ability of heat therapy to facilitate relaxation. I (Michael) recall taking annual vacations as a youth to a Christian retreat center in the mountains of Washington state, where we would take a sauna every evening, getting as hot as possible before diving into a snow bank or glacier-fed river. In retrospect, I can't say this is too safe for the cardiovascular system, but I surely did sleep well afterwards!

But heat can do a lot more than help you relax. Prior to the advent of antibiotics, heat was used in conventional medicine to treat infections, most notably syphilis.[26] But whole-body hyperthermia (WBH) is no longer a thing of the past. A database search of the National Library of Medicine yielded literally hundreds of articles on the use of hyperthermia just for cancer, including numerous clinical trials. A 2001 review by the Office of Alternative Medicine (OAM) at the National Institutes of Health (NIH) found good evidence that WBH was helpful in the treatment of cancer and encouraged further study.[27] Another review article found that hyperthermia significantly improved the prognosis of patients with rectal cancer when it was given in conjunction with chemotherapy and/or radiation. This applied to hyperthermia whether it was whole body or applied directly to the cancerous tissue. The authors particularly encouraged its use prior to surgery, since preoperative hyperthermia tended to shrink tumor size and make the cancer more resectable.[28]

While German researchers established the safety of whole-body hyperthermia,[29] it should be done carefully and in a controlled environment, particularly since some disease states, such as heart problems, multiple sclerosis, diabetes and high or low blood pressure, can be aggravated by heat.[30]

Sunlight has been proven to have several beneficial effects. Light converts melatonin, the sleep hormone, a depressant that causes a person to become tired and drowsy, into serotonin, a neurotransmitter that elevates energy and mood.[31] Therefore, high-intensity lights (e.g., 10,000 lux) are commonly recommended for patients struggling with depression, especially during the winter months when sunlight availability is greatly reduced.

Sunlight also promotes the production of vitamin D, as well as the breakdown of excess bilirubin. Premature newborns are commonly placed under "bili lights," because light triggers the conversion of bilirubin into a water-soluble form that can be excreted by the kidneys. The same thing could be accomplished by sunlight, although with the risk of overexposure and sunburn.

Therein lies the catch, sunshine is often blamed for damaging the skin and thereby causing cancer of the same. Is the criticism justified? Well, yes and no. Yes, sun damage to the skin is clearly related to basal cell and squamous cell skin cancers. But these are usually treated effectively with surgical removal.

However, the deadliest of skin cancers, melanoma, does not appear to be related to sun exposure. For example, the incidence of melanoma is five times higher in northern Scotland—where there is far less sun exposure—than in the Mediterranean islands. In Japan, 40 percent of melanomas occur on the soles of the feet. Since to our knowledge the Japanese do not sunbathe a great deal with their feet pointed toward the sky, sunshine is probably not the cause of this dreaded skin cancer.[32] In fact, sunlight may even protect against melanoma.[33] Rex Russell, M.D., author of *What the Bible Says About Healthy Living*, believes that there is another reason that the sun may be falsely accused. Poor nutrition renders the skin more vulnerable to sun-induced damage, and should therefore share the responsibility for problems like skin cancer.[34] The key to sun exposure appears to be balance: get plenty of sunlight, eat right and don't burn the skin.[35]

Detoxification. Due to its contention that illness is caused by an accumulation of toxins, detoxification has always played a central role in naturopathic therapeutics. While extended fasts between 7 and 21 days have been shown to lower cholesterol, good clinical trials of prolonged fasts testing their ability to detoxify the body and reverse disease are essentially nonexistent.[36] With regard to colon cleansing using either enemas (which can be self-administered and cleanse only the last part of the colon) or colonics (which are much more involved and require professional assistance), there is also a dearth of studies. Most citations in the medical literature are simply criticisms against their use on the basis that these practices are either dangerous, unproven or both.[37]

Evaluating Through the Grid of Spiritual Discernment

Several naturopathic concepts, such as autointoxication and the use of fasting, purging, diet, massage, herbs and meditation, appear to be closely related to central tenets of Eastern systems such as Ayurveda. Perhaps this is why naturopathic medicine has greeted Ayurveda, TCM and homeopathy with open arms. It is these latter associations that bear the greatest reason for spiritual concern, as we explain in their respective chapters. Another concern is that those patients who choose naturopathy as their primary medical system tend to become consumed with health issues, including concerns over the myriad of ways in which one can become exposed to toxins. Their diets and activities seem to become progressively more restrictive rather than leading them to freedom from disease and its concerns.

CONCLUSION

We see no conflict between Scripture and seeking to live in harmony with natural law through maintaining a proper diet, occasional fasting and having a reasonable awareness of threats to our health. But we do part ways with naturopathy when it embraces belief systems that are directly contrary to the teachings of Christ. That is the dimension of alternative medicine that Christians cannot accept.

Above all, keep a balanced perspective. If your government releases an advisory to boil your drinking water because excessive rains have overwhelmed the local water company's ability to maintain water purity, it is prudent to follow their advice. But don't become obsessed with toxin avoidance. It's like demons—you need to know they are around, but they should not preoccupy your thoughts.

For the kingdom of God is not meat and drink; but righteousness, and peace, and joy in the Holy Ghost (Rom. 14:17, *KJV*).

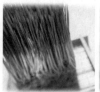

CHAPTER THIRTEEN

HOMEOPATHY

Homeopathy is "a system of therapeutics founded by Samuel Hahnemann (1755-1843) in which diseases are treated by drugs which are capable of producing in healthy persons symptoms similar to those of the disease to be treated, the drug being administered in minute doses."[1] In reference to his own theory of medicine, Samuel Hahnemann wrote, "The curative power of medicaments are derived from the fact they, in themselves, produce similar symptoms to those of the illness, and contain an energy superior to those in symptoms."[2]

EVALUATING THROUGH THE GRID OF HISTORY

Christian Frederick Samuel Hahnemann was born in Saxony, Germany, on April 10, 1755. A diligent student and gifted linguist, Samuel entered the study of medicine in 1777. He revealed his early ambitions when he wrote, "I shall read all the authors from Hippocrates up to the most recent, and the devil take us if I do not gather within my thoughts, the synthesis of knowledge, and be a great doctor who triumphs over death."[3] He supported himself by translating medical texts throughout medical school and attempted to start several private practices. While working on William Cullen's *Treatise on Materia Medica* in 1790, Hahnemann found himself disagreeing with Cullen's conclusion that the medicinal effect of cinchona (Peruvian bark from which quinine is derived) on malaria was due to its "tonic effect on the stomach."[4]

To test his idea, Hahnemann took a dose of cinchona (although he was perfectly healthy) and carefully observed its effects upon himself: coldness, drowsiness, thirst, heart palpitations, anxiety, prostration, headache, flushing, joint stiffness and bone pain. Since these were very similar to the symptoms he associated with malaria, Hahnemann proposed that cinchona (quinine) did not work by opposing the disease, because it produced symptoms similar to those of intermittent fever (malaria) in healthy people. He believed that those symptoms were not from the disease but from the body's attempt to rid itself of the illness.[5] Therefore, quinine (or any other remedy) was helpful only to the degree that it triggered symptoms similar to the illness that was being treated. He wrote:

> It is fundamentally important to understand that no differences exist between the manner of curing using the homeopathic remedy and the spontaneous and natural cure. To speak with greater propriety, what the remedy does is to excite the *"vis medicatrix,"* or rather, the process of natural cure; the medicine does not "cure" in itself or due to its mere presence, but rather by the vital reaction it provokes.[6]

In order to discover the symptoms or disease that remedies induced themselves, Hahnemann gave medicines to healthy volunteers—including himself—and recorded the symptoms they elicited in his reference manual, the *Materia Medica Pura*. When the sick presented themselves to Hahnemann, he took a detailed history of their symptoms and then searched the *Materia Medica* for the remedy whose symptom profile in healthy subjects most closely matched the symptoms being reported by the sick patient.[7]

He next discovered that he was able to get better results by giving lower doses of remedies. Instead of several grams of a drug, he gave milligrams. When he saw an improvement, he reduced the dosages further and further and further.

In 1810, Hahnemann published *The Organon of Rational Healing*, his first complete work detailing his new discoveries. Reaction from the orthodox medical community ranged from a general ho-hum to a few raging antagonists. He realized that in order for his newborn ideas to survive he would have to win over physicians before they had become entrenched in their own thinking. He returned to Leipzig where he sought and obtained a professorship at the University. There he proceeded to aggressively attack established medicine while promoting his new theory.[8]

The medicine of his day was an easy target. The standard treatments involved nothing less than what would be considered barbaric today. Rooted in

Greek humoralism (although the Greeks actually got the concept from Ayurvedic medicine), most treatments aggressively sought to rid the body of excess fluids (humors). Broussais (1772-1838), a Frenchman, vigorously advocated the use of leeches and venesections (draining the patient's blood). Hoffman (1742-1788) believed that degenerate acid humors must aggressively be eliminated from the body. For Stoll (1742-1788), bile was the culprit that needed to be purged through emetics (drugs to induce intense vomiting) or purgatives (drugs to induce fulminant diarrhea).

Today, in order to avoid side effects and toxicity, emphasis is placed on giving the lowest dose of medicine necessary to accomplish the therapeutic effect. But during Hahnemann's time, drugs were given in huge dosages, usually several grams at a time, because the toxic side effects were seen as necessary to the medicine accomplishing its purpose![9] The following is a poetic account of these primitive practices:

> This was the medicine; the patients died,
> And no one thought of asking who recovered.
> So 'mongst these hills and vales our hell-broths wrought
> More havoc, brought more victims to the grave
> By many than the pestilence had bought.
> To thousands I myself the poison gave:
> They pine and perished; I live on to hear
> Their reckless murderer's praises far and near.[10]

Hahnemann's method of lecturing was quite counterproductive. After reading a paragraph from his *Organon*, his professional calm and dignity would soon disappear and he would break out into a "raging hurricane" against the old methods and their practitioners.[11] One of his most devoted students wrote:

> Unfortunately the lectures were not fitted to win friends and followers for his theories or himself. For whenever possible, he poured forth a flood of abuse against the older medicine and its followers, with the result that his audience lessened every hour and finally consisted of only a few of his students. . . . Any others were present not for the subject matter but to hear the unfortunate method of presentation, so that their sense of humor might be freely tickled.[12]

Hahnemann had drawn a line in the sand, differentiating his own approach—which he dubbed homeopathy—from the conventional medicine of his day. The latter he named allopathy (a name that has stuck), since its goal was to oppose the illness with a remedy that was dissimilar. "Hahnemann purposely set down his principle in contrast to *contraria contrariis*, which was the only therapeutic method at that time, and which he therefore named 'Allopathy.'"[13]

Hahnemann left Leipzig for Koethen in 1821, where he spent the next 14 years practicing and writing as somewhat of a recluse. There he developed his theories on chronic diseases, publishing his first work devoted to the subject in 1828. In it, Hahnemann claimed that all chronic diseases (miasms) were due to one of three causes: (1) sycosis (fig-wart disease, i.e., gonorrhea), (2) syphilis (venereal chancre disease) or (3) psora (itch eruption, rashes). His chronic-disease theories aroused an additional violent reaction from the medical community, and many of his own disciples refused to follow him any longer.[14]

Two years later in 1830, his wife, Henriette, died and two of Hahnemann's surviving daughters moved in with him. There they lived together until 1834 when he met and married Marie Mélanie d'Hervilly of Paris. The 34 year-old French woman had journeyed from Paris to seek out the now-famous Hahnemann's help with her chronic abdominal pain. Within three days of her arrival, the 79-year-old Hahnemann had proposed to the young lady, 45 years his junior. The next year, Hahnemann took his bride and moved with her to Paris where he spent the final nine years of his life in a busy practice and social life, of which his Mélanie was an inseparable part. After a prolonged bout with bronchitis, Hahnemann died on the morning of July 2, 1843, at the age of 88. He was buried without a funeral in a grave with two other men. In 1898, his body was exhumed and removed to the famed Pére Lachaise Cemetery where a monument was eventually constructed in his honor.[15]

EVALUATING THROUGH THE GRID OF FAITH

Hahnemann was born into a Lutheran family and initially professed a belief in the God of the Bible, whom he claimed selected him to bring healing to mankind through the revelation of homeopathy. But other than church records for births, funerals and marriages, there is no evidence that Hahnemann ever attended worship. Furthermore, contrary to the Lutheran faith, it appears that Hahnemann rejected the claims of Christ. He is quoted as saying the principles of Confucius were higher than those of Christ, whom he called a "fervid emotionalist" and "Arch-Visionary."[16]

Hahnemann described himself as a Deist[17] and wrote to his second bride:

> The last sacrifice which it will be necessary to make for the sake of our union is to learn by heart the profession of the Protestant Lutheran faith in order to belong to the same cult as I. But you know, as I do myself, that these cults are clothes which one puts on or off only to accommodate oneself to the prejudices of the world.[18]

Hahnemann was a spiritual drifter. Detached from the Christian Church, he wandered through spiritualism into the occult.

> He advanced beyond [vitalism and the naturalism of Schelling and Hegel] to spiritualism and for a time lost his way in occultism . . . The essential material had to yield more and more ground and the purely spiritual (the dynamic) came more and more into the forefront. Hence we have in the end Hahnemann's outspoken tendency towards mesmerism.[19]

Homeopathic concepts seem to find their greatest compatibility with Eastern mysticism. Adolph Voegeli (a famous Swiss homeopath) believed that the best explanation for homeopathy comes from the Hindu *Sankhya philosophy*, which teaches that man has not only a physical body but an ethereal body with a special system of energetic channels.[20] Indeed, when I (Michael) sought the best books on homeopathy and biographies of Hahnemann, I had to order them from Delhi, India.

Homeopathic concepts seem to find their greatest compatibility with Eastern mysticism.

Undoubtedly, the philosophies which have counted, and still count, on the most followers in the entire homeopathic world, are those of pantheism and theosophy and both are doctrines whose adherents are most influential, being as they are, distinguished therapists.[21]

EVALUATING THROUGH THE
WHOLISTIC GRID

Homeopathy has four basic concepts or principles.

The Principle of Similars

Historians trace this concept's first use to Hindu sages in the tenth century B.C. The purpose of this principle is:

> To obtain a quick, easy and lasting cure, choose for every attack of illness a medicine which can produce a similar malady to the one it is to cure *(similia similibus curentur)*.[22]

Hippocrates affirmed this principle around 400 B.C. In the introduction to his *Organon*, Hahnemann quoted a student of Hippocrates as saying, "Illness arises by similar things and by similar things can the sick be made well. Vomiting can be made to cease by means of drugs used to stimulate vomiting."[23]

In the sixteenth century, Paracelsus restated this concept in his *Principle of Signatures*, which proposed that a diseased organ could be cured by a remedy that had a similar appearance in form or color. For example, curcuma was supposedly useful for jaundice because it was yellow.[24]

The Principal of Proving

In order to determine when a remedy should be used, it was necessary to know what symptoms it caused when given to a healthy patient. Healthy volunteers (usually fellow homeopaths) took therapeutic doses of common remedies and recorded the symptoms that they experienced. These were compiled and published in Hahnemann's *Materia Medica Pura*.[25] Since Hahnemann believed that the patient's illness should be treated with a substance that induced a similar illness, Hahnemann prescribed a remedy whose list of reported symptoms most closely matched those for which the patient was seeking relief. The lists of symptoms for some of these remedies are incredibly long. For example, *belladonna* (nightshade) has 1,422 symptoms; *nux vomica* (vomit nut) has 1,267. With so many possible symptoms, one wonders how useful such a list could actually be.[26]

The Principle of the Single Remedy

Hahnemann believed that a single remedy should be used at any given time. He strongly opposed the mixing of remedies and would blast with harsh criticism anyone who dared to do so.

The Principle of Potentiation (Dynamisation)

"There is a remedy for every disease," says Paracelsus. "The less the quantity, the greater the effect."[27] As Hahnemann continued to experiment, he used progressively smaller doses, believing that the greater the dilution, the greater the potency. He attributed this to dynamisation. Also known as potentiation, this method first involved thorough triturating (grinding) of the original remedy into a fine powder. A predetermined amount (such as one grain) of this powder was placed in nine drops of a solvent, such as water or alcohol. The mixture was then shaken vigorously (referred to as succussion by Hahnemann). Then this 1:10 dilution (one part original and nine parts solvent, also referred to as 1X) was diluted again, taking one drop of the 1:10 solution, combining it with nine drops of fresh solvent and succussing it to make a 1:100 or 2X ($1x10^{-2}$) solution. In order to make a 6X ($1x10^{-6}$) solution, this process was repeated four more times. To make a 12X solution, it was repeated 10 more times.[28]

If Hahnemann desired a 6X solution, why did he not just put one drop of active remedy into 999,999 drops of solvent and shake that up? Because he believed that there was more to the process than simple dilution. Hahnemann reasoned that the trituration and succussion process released dynamic energy (i.e., vital force, a spiritual discernment) from the remedy into the homeopathic solution. Therefore, the more the succussion, and the more dilute the substance, the more potent Hahnemann believed it to be.

Obviously homeopathic medicine is not wholistic, because one tiny particle solves all.

EVALUATING THROUGH THE GRID OF SCIENCE

Hahnemann did the best he could to develop a health-disease-therapeutics model that would be superior to the prevailing medicine of his day. All biases aside—with his emphasis on proper hygiene and his rejection of bloodlettings, blisters and toxic dosages of medications—he probably succeeded. Since his time, medicine has come to side with Hahnemann on many of the objections that he had to endure regarding what was practiced 200 years ago.[29]

- He was one of the first to oppose the barbaric practices of his day: venesection, leeches, blistering agents, etc.
- He pushed strongly for the prevention of epidemics (which he recognized early on as having a germ origin) through improved cleanliness, hygiene and proper diet.
- Largely as a result of his efforts, the medical profession reconsidered its practice of prescribing huge dosages of drugs. Modern-day allopathic prescriptions, in milligrams or micrograms, are similar to some of the early homeopathic low potencies.[30]

Dr. Johannes Hadick confessed quite frankly, "Medicine as approved by the State does not realize how homeopathical it has become in one century." Proofs of this are evident and frequently quite apparent to the laymen: dry-cupping, leeches, bloodletting, regular purging and laxatives are known to patients nowadays only from hearsay. The large medicinal bottles and medicine mixtures of our grandfathers' and great grandfathers' times have disappeared. The doses of remedies administered have become smaller and smaller in medicinal contents. In many cases, they have reached the smallness of homeopathic doses.[31]

- He was the first to systematically study and record the effects of drugs.
- His methods of vigorous grinding and succussion probably improved the absorption of medicines.

But that was then. Today, Hahnemann and modern medicine would still find very little ground for agreement. For one thing, Hahnemann's views on disease causality are totally incompatible with the current Western biomedical model.

The Causes of Disease

Let's consider the example of diabetes. We understand today that islet cells of the pancreas make insulin, and that the islet cells have been destroyed in someone who develops juvenile onset diabetes. They cannot produce their own insulin, and so, in order to survive, they need to take insulin by injection. But to treat juvenile diabetes in a manner consistent with homeopathic philosophy, a homeopath would search the homeopathic reference manual for a remedy which, when given by mouth to a healthy person, causes bad breath, excessive thirst, urination and weight loss. But insulin does not do this when given to a healthy person.

To summarize, homeopathic theory is an entirely different conceptual framework for the diagnosis and treatment of disease. It requires near-total rejection of anatomy, physiology and biochemistry as we know it. What would a conscientious homeopath do today for an insulin-dependent diabetic? He would probably refer the patient to the local allopath for proper diabetic management.

Provings

Provings, including Hahnemann's cinchona experience, have not been reproduced by nonhomeopaths. In a famous lecture series given in 1842 by Oliver Wendell Holmes, M.D., the renowned Harvard professor cited numerous independent investigators who tested cinchona and other remedies, but without the results claimed by homeopaths. Obviously, the homeopaths disagree, but supporting evidence is extremely scant.[32]

Infinitesimal Dilutions

According to Avogadro's hypothesis, once a solute is diluted past 6.23×10^{-23}, there are no molecules of active ingredient left in the solution. Therefore, it seems truly implausible that a remedy could have any legitimate effect after it has been diluted past that point (i.e., greater than 24X or 12C). But by the time of his death, Hahnemann was convinced that his most potent and effective remedy was two "sniffs" of a 30C solution (that is one cc of original ingredient in 999,999,999,999,999,999,999,999,999,999,999,999,999,999,999,999,999, 999,999 cc of solvent).[33] In a double-blind 1993 study done at the University of Freiburg, 45 healthy volunteers were unable to tell whether or not they were taking a placebo or homeopathic belladonna 30C.[34] Although one would naturally tend to think that any effect of such an extreme dilution could only be attributed to the placebo effect, others claim otherwise.[35] Individuals are often exposed to homeopathic substances in greater concentrations as they occur naturally, such as in our foods (e.g., calcarea, silicea, carbonicum) than in the homeopathic remedies themselves, with no perceivable effect.[36]

Research

"There is no scientific explanation for the mechanism of action of homeopathic medicines, although there are several theories."[37] Despite 200 years of existence, no one has been able to propose and adequately validate a satisfactory mechanism for homeopathic medicines. While there are several theories (such as the remedy making an energy imprint on the water in which it is dissolved), none have been proven to any sufficient degree. This is acknowledged by homeopaths themselves. At the 1996 World Congress on Complementary Medicine, the director of research of the Royal London Homeopathic Hospital said, in effect, "We know homeopathy works. We just don't know how."[38]

Clinical Trials

But does it really work? Table 1 in appendix B shows several clinical trials, including the year the study was published, the principal author, the number of participants in the study, the remedies being tested, the problem being treated and whether or not the homeopathic remedies were concluded to be more effective than placebo. Please refer to table B-1 for a detailed account. However, if you have little scientific background and merely want to know if homeopathy worked, just take our word for it that 8 out of the 11 trials did not help the patient. On a larger scale, Kleijnen reviewed 107 controlled trials and reported that while most trials were of "very low quality," there were many exceptions, and the results showed a trend in favor of homeopathy.[39] On the other hand, Edward Ernst, professor of complementary medicine at the University of Exeter, concluded:

> Of the trials conducted into the effects of homeopathy since 1991, it is clear that most with good methodology give negative results and those with poor methodology give results in favor of homeopathy.[40]

In other words, when research studies are designed well, they tend to conclude that homeopathy has little if any benefit—hardly proof of Hahnemann's contention that he would eventually conquer disease and triumph over death itself.[41]

EVALUATING THROUGH THE GRID OF SPIRITUAL DISCERNMENT

Jesus said, "By their fruits ye shall know them" (Matt. 7:20, *KJV*). That being the case, we should have serious concern regarding the use of homeopathy, because the fruit that is produced is not good.

Hahnemann's Personal Life

Even according to those who were closest to him, Hahnemann was prideful, abrasive and reclusive. Other than his wife, it seemed that he had no genuine friends.

> His wooing of supporters to his idea was impetuous and incessant, but he almost hated his adherents. There is much talk of his ever-increasing rudeness, of sudden breaches of old friendship, of unforeseen and unrestrained attacks on his advocates. As a doctor, he followed the complaints and maladies of his patients to the last accessible corner, but as a teacher he shut himself up within an impregnable wall of obstinacy. Any opposition invariably drove him into sharper formulations, and led him to step up his doctrine to such an extent that it ultimately became incomprehensible and unacceptable even to his most fervent votaries. Thus he fanatically destroyed the bridges between his own mind and others'.[42]

The tale of his children is that of one tragedy after another, almost as if his household was cursed.

> In 1830, when Hahnemann was 75 years old, his wife died in Koethen. Of his eleven children, only two remained, both widowed daughters. The others had all died by suicide, murder or other tragic causes or had disappeared.[43]

His two remaining daughters, Luise and Charlotte, lived together in a house Hahnemann bought for them prior to his departure to Paris. Neighbors reported that they both suffered from intense phobias, sleeping only a few hours during the day and remaining up all night for fear something evil might happen to them. They installed a bellpull in the house and rang it on the landing every half hour to show that they were still awake.[44]

Homeopathy as a "BeachHead" for Occult Activity

In his book *Healing at Any Price*, Pfeiffer warns against the employment of homeopathy, particularly if the practitioner is using substances more dilute than 6X or 12X in potency, or if the practitioner utilizes or speaks of (psychic) energy, pendulums, palmistry, magnetism or healing at a distance. As a former homeopath and psychic healer who is now a Christian, Pfeiffer warns that some homeopaths add magic to their remedies to increase their effectiveness. Such a remedy "can serve as a beachhead for the enemy and can lead to occult oppression."[45] There are reports of those whose physical symptoms cleared up with homeopathy, but psychological and spiritual problems developed in the lives of the patients and their families.

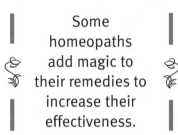

> Some homeopaths add magic to their remedies to increase their effectiveness.

This is what I (Michael) have repeatedly observed in families who have made homeopathy a central focus of their lives. A pattern of events seems to often take place.

1. A parent, usually the mother, is concerned for her family's health.
2. Finding insufficient answers in allopathic medicine, she discovers homeopathy.
3. After some initial success with homeopathic remedies (for example, she can't get her child's fever to come down with acetaminophen or ibuprofen, but it finally responds to a homeopathic remedy), she becomes convinced of the effectiveness of homeopathy.
4. She purchases a homeopathic home kit and uses it whenever illness strikes. Doctors are only consulted when absolutely necessary (i.e., the child is still sick despite her best efforts).
5. From a presumably objective physician's view, they are the sickest family in the church (or in the practice). In other words, despite the fact that they are convinced that they are utilizing the most effective medical system, the overall health of their family seems to be sliding downhill. They seem to be caught up in a great delusion.
6. When the family renounces their use of homeopathy, their physical and spiritual health seems to improve dramatically.

The Necessity of Faith

Some have suggested that homeopathic remedies may have a medicinal effect, but only for people who believe in them. That is essentially the placebo effect, but it also is a New Age concept of belief (i.e., believe hard enough and it will become true). For example, after beginning to question the basis for his homeopathic practice, Dr. Donner tested 4X-12X potencies versus placebo in a blinded fashion on volunteer patients. Neither placebos nor homeopathic remedies produced any change in subjects who did not believe in homeopathy. On the other hand, believers in homeopathy had numerous—even violent— symptoms, even when given a placebo. One homeopathic doctor got such fierce migraine attacks that she could only work part-time for a year after taking a placebo for three days.

It is this misunderstanding of faith that appears to be pivotal as to whether or not an individual practicing homeopathy (or, for that matter, many other therapies) develops evidence of occult involvement. If someone walks into a health-food store and purchases a homeopathic remedy, thinking it is an herbal preparation, there does not seem to be any adverse effect spiritually. There is no transfer of faith. However, if they place their faith in healing or protection from disease into homeopathy, adverse spiritual circumstances seem to follow.

> Man is a spiritual being and only the spirit can heal the body. Illness only exists because the spirit of man considers that illness can exist. By presenting to the spirit (or vital force) the correct medicine in the correct dose for the correct period of time, the spirit changes its considerations, and the illness is gone. Curative homeopathic medicines are seldom used in a material form. Healing energy is released from the medicinal substance through the separation of its particles by an inert medium, during the application of physical energy. The healing energy specific in quality in accordance with its material source, has a direct action on the vital force. Homeopathic medicines probably have no direct action upon the physical body of the organism.[46]

CONCLUSION

In reaction to the horrible medical practices of his day, Samuel Hahnemann developed a disease and therapeutics model that shows striking similarities to concepts promoted by Hippocrates and Paracelsus and finds a comfortable fit in a Hindu religious paradigm. This model proposes that toxic substances possess energies that are released into solution when they are progressively diluted to infinitesimal doses. These diluted remedies are believed to cure the illness by producing a disease that is similar to the one being treated and, thereby, provoking the body to throw off the disease.

There is evidence that homeopathy was more effective than the standard medicine of 200 years ago, probably due to the innocuous nature of its remedies compared to the extremely harsh and toxic allopathic modalities. However, while orthodox medicine made advances over the next centuries, homeopathy did not. Today, despite considerable research, there is very little evidence to support homeopathy.

Furthermore, its claims run completely contrary to generally accepted principles of science and logic. Homeopathy simply does not fit with natural law. To accept that an infinitesimally diluted substance has disease-treating effects would mean that fundamental principles of modern physics and biochemistry are false.

The biography of its founder, the mystical associations of many of its practitioners and the testimony of some who have come out of homeopathy serve as stern warnings that homeopathy, particularly in its use of high dilutions, should be shunned.

Death has no further power over man, the homeopaths have taken away his sting! For, if shaking and rubbing a dead medicinal substance, reduced to an unimaginable size, can give an effective power passing all comprehension, surely nobody can be surprised if he sees dead men brought to life by shaking and rubbing, sustained appropriately.[47]

Hahnemann never conquered death, Jesus did. Our health is very much dependent upon who or what we trust.

CHAPTER FOURTEEN

TRADITIONAL CHINESE MEDICINE (TCM)

EVALUATING THROUGH THE GRID OF HISTORY

Traditional Chinese medicine (TCM) includes several therapeutic approaches, the most well-known being acupuncture. A careful study of available textbooks and records indicates that "there is no reference to acupuncture (as a therapeutic method in any Chinese text before 90 B.C., and . . . the oldest existing text to discuss medical practices that faintly resemble current Chinese medicine dates from the end of the third century B.C."[1]

Despite the fact that this coincides precisely with the birth of Taoism, legend traces TCM to Huang Di, the Yellow Emperor, who supposedly gained his knowledge through contact with the dead. Legend has it that his teachings were passed down by word-of-mouth for 2,000 years, until around 200 B.C., when the *Yellow Emperor's Inner Classic (Huang Di Nei Jing)* text was compiled. During the next several centuries, Chinese medicine grew in its influence and became more systemized. However, after the Qing dynasty opened China to the West, TCM suffered such a serious setback that "in 1822, acupuncture was formally eliminated from the Imperial Medical College."[2] Eventually, TCM experienced resurgence in the 1900s.

EVALUATING THROUGH THE GRID OF FAITH

Taoism originated in China around 300 B.C. during a time marked by great strife and political upheaval (the Warring States period). This philosophy arose in part out of a reaction to Confucianism, which taught that "people can live a good life only in a well-disciplined society that stresses attention to ceremony, duty and public service. In contrast, the Taoist ideal was a person who avoids conventional social obligations and leads a simple, spontaneous, and meditative life close to nature."[3]

There are four premises found in Taoism that underlie TCM.

Premise 1: Yin and Yang

According to the religion that arose out of this philosophy, Tao, "the way of the universe," is the "first-cause" or cosmic force behind nature's order (a personal creator is not the first cause but an impersonal force). Tao has two faces, yin and yang, which oppose each other, yet are one. They are always present simultaneously. Just as seasons change, one flows from the other. Their original meaning appears to have come from the "shady and sunny sides of a hill." The sunlit southern side, with its plants and animals that prefer it, are yang, while the northern side is yin. Thus, yin represents fall and winter and that which is dark, cold, slow, feminine and so on. Yang represents spring and summer, light, warmth, speed, masculinity, etc. There are five hollow yin organs and five solid yang organs. Each yin organ is paired with a yang organ, and each of these pairs is linked with one of the five phases (see premise 2). Human beings are said to be inseparable from yin, yang and the world about them. In this system, there is no absolute good or evil, just balance or imbalance, harmony or disharmony.[4]

Premise 2: Five Phases

Another major premise in Chinese medicine is that of the five phases (*wu xing*). Similar to Ayurveda, the five phases are earth, metal, water, wood and fire. These five phases are correlated with the five yin and yang organs. The ancient Chinese believed that virtually all health and disease phenomena moved in these relationships. Thus, they explained the cause (and treatment) of disease from an entirely different perspective—one of which is quite mystical—involving planets and energy relationships unknown outside Eastern philosophy.

Premise 3: Qi

According to Taoism, qi (also spelled ch'i or ki and pronounced "chee") is the life force that pervades the body and "causes most physiological functions and maintains the health and vitality of the individual. Qi is sometimes compared to wind captured in a sail; we cannot observe the wind directly, but we can infer its presence as it fills the sail. In a similar fashion, the movements of the body and the movement of substances within the body are all signs of the action of qi."[5]

Qi supposedly moves throughout the body via channels (also called meridians), going first through an internal organ (viscera) and then across the body's surface to connect with the channel of a related organ. Points along the body surface function as valves or regulators, providing access to and control of the qi that is traveling through the channel. There has been considerable debate within the Chinese community as to the number of channels and locations of acupuncture points along them.

According to Taoism, when qi energy flows unhindered between man and the universe, good health is the result. Illness occurs if qi becomes hindered or blocked. "Ultimately, all illness is a disturbance of qi within the body."[6]

Premise 4: Microcosm

Taoism proclaims that man is a microcosm of the universe, which is the macrocosm. In other words, man is an image of the universe (contrary to the biblical view that sees man as created in the image of God, the creator of the universe). Thus, man is one with the universe, and one can effect a change in the universe through humanity, and conversely. This explains the significant emphasis on astrology in ancient China.

In a similar fashion, it is believed that any organ of the human body can serve as a microcosm of the whole person. Therefore, one can examine the eye and see the entire person (iridology), or the foot (reflexology), or the ear (auriculotherapy), or the hand (*Koryo sooji chim*, a Korean variation) and so on. Since the entire body is manifested in a single organ or region, one can treat the entire body from that location with needles, pressure, magnets, etc.

EVALUATING THROUGH THE WHOLISTIC GRID

Since all disease is believed to be caused by a disruption in the flow of qi, the TCM practitioner diagnoses the cause of illness on the basis of where qi is blocked. He or she does this through taking a medical history, examining the patient (spirit, form, bearing, head, face, body excretions, and the color, shape, markings and coating of the tongue, and then listening to the speech and smelling the breath, body and excreta) and palpating the pulses.

Acupuncturists believe there are 12 pulses—six in each wrist—one for each of the 12 meridians. "The pulse is divided into three parts: the middle part is adjacent to the styloid process of the radius, in what is called the 'bar position.' The styloid is the pointed bone felt on the outside border of the wrist in the radial pulse area when the palms are facing up. The inch is distal to it and the cubit is proximal."[7] Each one of these three points is palpated for a superficial and deep pulse. Thus, despite the fact that there is only one radial artery present, the Oriental practitioner is somehow able to derive six pulses, one for each of the six meridians that are said to traverse the wrist.

Once again, notice the striking similarity to Ayurveda. It makes us wonder if these concepts—along with many in Taoism—did not originate in India, since it was around 200-300 B.C. that not only Taoism and TCM apparently began but Buddhism was brought from India to China.

Normalizing Qi: Traditional Chinese Approaches

Once the site(s) of obstructed energy flow has been identified, the TCM practitioner employs any of several Chinese treatments developed for the purpose of accessing the patient's qi and normalizing its flow. These approaches include acupressure, moxibustion, Chinese herbal medicine, diet and qigong.

1. **Acupuncture.** When using acupuncture, a thin needle is inserted into points that are believed to be culprits in the illness. The practitioner then attempts to sense the arrival of qi at that point. The essential aim of the acupuncturist is to obtain qi at the needling site. The physician seeks either an objective or subjective indication that the qi has arrived. Qi can become manifest to the practitioner through sensations experienced by the hands as the needle is manipulated, through observation or through reports from the patient. The sensation of the arrival of qi often is felt by the practitioner as a gentle grasping of the needle at the site, as if one is fishing, and one's line has suddenly been seized by the fish. The patient senses the arrival of qi as a sensation of itching, numbness, soreness or a swollen feeling. The patient might experience local temperature changes or a distinct "electrical sensation."[8]

2. **Acupressure.** Also known as shiatsu or g-jo, acupressure is based upon the same concepts as acupuncture, but instead of needles, one uses pressure over the meridian points.

3. **Moxibustion.** Also known as jiu fa, moxibustion "refers to the burning of the dried and powdered leaves of artemesia vulgaris (ai ye), either on or in proximity to the skin, in order to affect the movement of qi in the channel, locally or at a distance."[9]

4. **Cupping and Bleeding.** Reminiscent of humoralism and Western medicine just a couple of centuries ago, TCM still employs mechanical efforts to improve local circulation. In cupping, a vacuum is induced in a small glass or bamboo cup, which is then applied to the skin surface. The purpose is to drain or remove cold and damp evils from the body or to assist blood circulation. Bleeding may be utilized to drain a channel or to remove heat from the body.

5. **Chinese Herbal Medicine.** Also known as Zhong Yao, chinese herbal medicine is not a new way of practicing medicine. The Chinese, like virtually every human culture, have employed herbs extensively for medicinal purposes. However, the philosophy upon which China's traditional herbal medicine is practiced is based upon the ancient doctrines of qi, the five phases and so on. Therefore, diseases, symptoms and herbal effects are all interpreted in the context of these beliefs. For example, *Ma huang* is an herb that contains ephedra. The scientific explanation for its ability to open up clogged nasal passages is based upon its ability to stimulate receptors on blood vessels, causing them to constrict. But the TCM practitioner would explain the same observations as the body throwing off damp evils and restoring the unimpeded flow of qi.

6. **Qigong.** Pronounced "chee goong," qigong balances the body's qi, not with needles, but with an inner force accessed through mental and breathing exercises. While qigong has been practiced in the Orient for centuries, its popularity soared in the 1980s in response to two highly publicized cases heralding its success. In the first, a prominent 21-year-old athlete was cured of lung cancer through practicing a walking form of qigong (guo lin gong fa) for 10-14 hours per day. In the second, a 36-year-old factory worker had been paralyzed for seven months in the wake of an accident that had

fractured his skull and spine. After six consecutive hours of treatment by a qigong master who was 10 miles away, the paraplegic worker was able to walk with crutches. Two months later, he was walking with only a slight limp.[10]

There are two different ways in which qigong is practiced. In the first, the patient tries to balance their own qi through deep breathing and relaxation. In the second, a qigong master does it for them. A master is an individual who has learned how to build up his own personal qi to the extent that he or she can give it to others.[11]

Qigong is claimed to be beneficial in a wide variety of disease states, including (but not limited to) allergy, asthma, cancer, circulation problems, deafness, diabetes, headache, hormone problems, hypertension, injuries, kidney, liver disease, lung problems and stroke.

EVALUATING THROUGH THE GRID OF SCIENCE

At a 1996 Washington, D.C., conference on alternative medicine, experts from China taught on TCM. Through interpreters, they explained the basis for TCM—the Taoist concepts of qi, yin and yang, and so on (i.e., religion, not science). The Chinese, throughout a majority of their history, have not conducted scientific studies on TCM. Because the basis of TCM is in their Taoist religion, the Chinese assumed TCM to be true. They never saw any need for scientific study. But it is Westerners who have embraced TCM who are looking for scientific validation.

Problems with Acupuncture Point Selection

TCM maintains that qi meridians are well-defined, as is evidenced by charts depicting these channels. However, acupuncture points are frequently selected based upon the fact that they are tender and have no relationship whatsoever to recognized meridians.

In some cases, points that do not lie on specific channels or form part of the collection of recognized extra points can be identified by their tenderness. These points are known as *ah shi,* or "ouch, that's it," points, and are an important part of clinical acupuncture's traditional history and contemporary practice.[12]

This raises a serious question. If acupuncture is truly working to correct the disruption in qi as it flows through channels, how does one explain the necessity or effectiveness of treating the patient where no channel is even acknowledged to exist? There are only two possibilities. First, there is a channel traversing there, but after 2,000 and more years of practice, we just don't know it. Second, the premise is false. We are not really treating channels or qi. There is a different mechanism by which acupuncture exerts any effect. We propose the latter.

The most likely explanation for the possible benefit of acupuncture has nothing to do with meridians or qi. Some studies have demonstrated that piercing the skin with a needle at certain points stimulates nerve pathways to the brain involved with pain relief.[13] Others show that it may affect the activity of the autonomic nervous system, causing changes such as a slowing of the heart rate.[14] "Counterirritation" describes the concept that pressure or irritation of a point (unrelated to acupuncture points) can result in a reduction of pain or a sense of numbness or pain elsewhere. When certain "trigger points" are pressed, needled or anesthetized, sensations can increase or diminish at remote locations. These points are believed to occur via neurological reflexes, in which nerve impulses from the stimulated muscle go to the spinal cord where they then interact with nerves supplying the referred areas. Ronald Melzack of McGill University discovered that there was a 70 percent correlation between acupuncture points and known trigger points.[15]

Frank Chapman, one of the first osteopathic physicians, discovered and taught about somatovisceral reflexes—also known as Chapman's reflexes—in which he claimed that pressure points in the skin can, when stimulated, reflexively affect internal organs which have a related nerve supply.[16] There are also reflexes known to occur in muscles (such as described by Janet Travell, M.D.) and ligaments or joints. For example, when the iliolumbar ligament (ILL) is injured, it tends to refer pain into the groin on the same side. Thus, if a person has a back problem but presents with groin pain, an anesthetic injected into an injured ILL in the back will often result in relief of the groin pain.[17] Once again, these mechanisms have nothing to do with qi or meridians.

Clinical Studies

Since acupuncture came to the West in the 1970s, it has been subjected to literally hundreds of research studies. However, there are only a few with reliable results that validate its theory and practice. While individual studies occasionally appear to be supportive, they are often discredited by other researchers who conclude that the studies were poorly designed and inconclusive.

For example, in a 1989 review of 14 studies that used randomized and controlled trials of acupuncture to treat chronic pain, one researcher concluded that acupuncture was better than placebo and conventional treatment. But a second meta-analysis of 51 studies the next year disagreed.[18]

A 1990 study utilizing acupuncture to treat tennis elbow showed that acupuncture patients did better early on than superficially needled patients. But there was no difference between the two groups at 3 and 12 months after treatment.[19] A 1991 review of 13 trials treating asthma with acupuncture concluded that it had no proven benefit in this condition.[20]

In 1998, while acknowledging their concerns regarding the research quality, a consensus panel of the National Institutes of Health summarized its review of acupuncture studies. They concluded that there was good evidence that acupuncture can reduce nausea and vomiting after chemotherapy and surgery and pain after dental procedures. They also concluded that acupuncture could be helpful for several other conditions, such as headaches, provided that it was combined with other treatment modalities.[21] But from a quality of research perspective, the bottom line was summarized in a complementary medicine textbook which said, "Disappointingly little has been achieved by literally hundreds of attempts to evaluate acupuncture. Major methodological flaws are apparent in the vast majority of studies."[22] (See table B-2 for a complete summary on a number of acupuncture studies published in recent years.)

Qigong Research

Recalling that there are two methods of qigong, there appear to be at least two mechanisms of action, one physiological and the other psychic or spiritual. In regard to a physical action, beneficial effects can be gained by increasing the oxygenation of tissues through improved breathing. Other beneficial effects may be obtained through relaxation. One researcher placed asthma patients on 16 weeks of deep diaphragmatic breathing exercises. Patients were able to greatly reduce their asthma medications and intensity of asthma symptoms. They were also able to increase their physical activity level nearly 300 percent during the study period. (However, many patients returned to their sedentary lifestyle and original medication levels just two months later).[23] Similarly, patients who had emphysema were able to significantly improve their lung function through training in breathing techniques.[24] More specific to qigong itself is a study involving 123 patients with various types of cancer. Those who added qigong exercises to their conventional medication showed greater improvements in strength, appetite, weight gain and immune system function parameters when compared to controls. Their regimen involved qigong exercises for at least two hours daily for three to six months.[25]

There have also been numerous studies documenting that energy is emitted from qigong masters in a variety of ways. Most often, the increase in energy is emitted from the qigong master's hands and is several times greater than that measured from controlled individuals, or from the same qigong masters when they are not in the "qigong state."[26] Zhang measured unique changes in the brain waves of qigong masters when they were in the qigong state.[27]

> Emitted Qi is defined as energy that is emitted from the body of a Qigong master—generally, but not necessarily, from the hand—when the master is in the "Qigong state." In most cases, the master holds his or her hand above an object or person and concentrates on emitting energy to the object.[28]

What has this emitted energy been able to do? In a Chinese study, an average of 25 percent of human stomach cancer cells in a culture dish were either killed or inactivated when treated with emitted qi for one hour. No effect was seen on control cells. Similar results were obtained with human uterine cancer cells.[29] A researcher demonstrated beneficial effects in cancerous mice and recommended qigong be added to chemotherapy regimens.[30] In a study involving 18 pigs that were given a spinal cord injury resulting in paraplegia, 11 out of the 12 pigs treated with emitted qi were able to walk again, while all six of the controls remained paralyzed. Beneficial effects have been demonstrated in the cardiovascular system, in T-lymphocytes and in hypersensitivity reactions.[31] The following statement makes an incredible claim for the emission of qi:

The effects of emitted qi have been demonstrated in many ways. Its application in human studies has been followed by improvement in many medical conditions, including the function of the immune system. In animal studies, emitted qi has altered heart rates and slowed the growth rate of induced cancers. In clinical laboratory experiments, emitted qi has been shown to kill bacteria and viruses progressively as the time of exposure to emitted qi increases. In agricultural studies, the germination rate of rice and wheat seeds has increased or decreased according to the intent of the Qigong master. In the physics laboratory, emitted qi has been reported to alter the physical properties of matter.[32]

However, at least when it comes to humans, it appears that the power behind qigong may be nullified if the patient does not truly believe in it. In a controlled study, Wirth compared qigong with therapeutic touch (TT) using EMG (electromyography—measurements of muscle activity). Patients were divided into three groups: (1) those who were already seeing a qigong practitioner; (2) those who were already seeing a TT practitioner; and (3) those who believed in neither. Patients receiving and believing in qigong showed the greatest response to qigong. The TT patients showed a milder, less significant change. But those who disbelieved in either process showed no measurable change in muscle activity from either approach.[33]

EVALUATING THROUGH THE GRID OF SPIRITUAL DISCERNMENT

While the scientific basis (or lack of it) for TCM should raise some questions as to its validity, the potential interaction with the spiritual realm is of even greater concern.

Pulse Diagnosis

In TCM, strong emphasis is placed on the practitioners' need to tune in to what the qi is telling them as they take their clients' pulses. Since there is only one artery in the area in which there are claimed to be six pulses, one has to wonder just what the practitioner of Oriental medicine is actually feeling. One author wrote:

When he (the practitioner) palpates at each position, at each level he quite deliberately, silently, says to himself, "I am now listening to the pulse of the small intestine (for example), to hear and to try and under-stand what it is saying to me. This almost ritual approach to the reading of pulses has often been sneered at by Westerners who understand so lit-tle of Far East wisdom. It does not matter if it takes a whole hour to feel and to access the pulses. It is important to cultivate the ability to listen to the vital message that will become clearly revealed to the calm and receptive mind. What is the Life Force doing in each of the Organs and Organ Meridians? The human being will tell you through the pulses, the inmost secrets of the Life Force animating it—and its message will be a truthful message. If the practitioner is sincere and genuinely seeks to understand and receive the message, it will be there. Accept what you read—whether your reasoning tells you it ought to be different or not. It is not up to the practitioner to dictate to the pulses what message they "ought" to be giving and therefore only listen to what he thinks the mes-sage should be. The practitioner's task is to read the message as the Life Force in the patient who gives it. . . . Never neglect the pulses. Even if you are not "acting on the pulse signs," see what the pulses have to say.[34]

Obviously, the assessment of qi is neither scientific nor objective. Since the concept of qi is inconsistent with Scripture, since it has never truly been estab-lished as a distinct physical reality by science, since pulse diagnosis is very sub-jective in nature and since it appears that the examiner must involve himself in what appears to be a psychic practice, it seems very plausible that pulse diagno-sis enters into the realm of the occult. This is not surprising given the fact that Taoism has always been linked with the occult.

Qigong's Psychic/Occult Nature

The psychic or occult activity of qigong becomes rather obvious when one reads of accounts such as the "long-distance" healings noted at the beginning of this section. Some studies have documented emitted qi from up to 1,200 miles away with effects similar to those noted at close range.[35] One researcher reports:

Since the late 1980's the principal author has succeeded in storing (+) Qi Gong energy on a variety of substances including small sheets of paper, and recently has been able to intensify this energy by concen-trating it as it passes through a cone-shaped, tapered glass or plastic object placed directly on the (+) Qi Gong energy stored paper. Application of (+) Qi Gong energy stored paper on the cardio-vascular representation area of the medulla oblongata at the occipital area of the skull often improved circulation and enhanced drug uptake.[36]

However, with striking similarity to that which has been reported by psychics, the researcher goes on to note that utilizing such power has its consequences.

This direct method often results in the practitioner developing intestinal micro-hemorrhage within 24 hours which may or may not be noticed as mild intestinal discomfort with soft, slightly tarry stool.[37]

As one would expect if the occult were involved, patients practicing qigong have reported a variety of bizarre experiences. One report states that 109 cases of mental disorders were a result of qigong, including 47 with schizophrenia and 62 with neurosis.[38] Mental and psychological problems have occurred with enough frequency that they are now referred to as qigong deviation syndrome.

Patients experienced warmness, chilliness, itching . . . numbness, soreness, bloatedness, relaxation, tenseness, floating, dropping, enlargement or constriction of the body image, a sensation of rising to the sky, falling off, standing upside down, playing on the swing following respiration, circulation of the intrinsic Qi, electric shock . . . dreamland illusions, unreality and pseudohallucination. These phenomena were transient and vanished as the exercise terminated. Qigong deviation syndrome has become a diagnostic term and is now used widely in China.[39]

CONCLUSIONS

False Religion

Taoism and Christianity are totally incompatible with one another. According to Scripture, man is created in the image of God, not in the image of the universe. While Taoism speaks of impersonal yin and yang, Scripture identifies a world of good and evil spirits. Taoism claims that man can regain health and immortality through personal disciplines and the practice of magic, alchemy and TCM.

Scripture condemns interaction with the occult, requires our obedience to God's natural and spiritual law and affirms what we all know to be true—that the

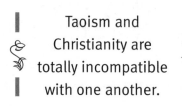

Taoism and Christianity are totally incompatible with one another.

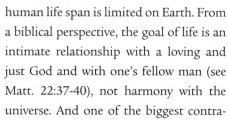

human life span is limited on Earth. From a biblical perspective, the goal of life is an intimate relationship with a loving and just God and with one's fellow man (see Matt. 22:37-40), not harmony with the universe. And one of the biggest contra-

dictions between the two religions is that Taoism proclaims itself as the way, when Jesus said, "I am the way, and the truth, and the life; no one comes to the Father, but through Me" (John 14:6).

Faulty Approach

TCM is based upon an ancient, limited and error-filled understanding of anatomy and physiology. Two thousand years ago, the medical profession embraced extremely flawed concepts regarding a variety of biological functions, including blood circulation, the purpose and function of numerous organs, the existence and role of microscopic organisms and so on. Many of these misconceptions were only resolved in the last 300 years. However, TCM still embraces such errors, including organs that do not exist (such as the *triple warmer,* which still has a wrist pulse for diagnosis) and bases its entire practice upon concepts that are totally incompatible with known facts.

Faulty Science

Acupuncture may work physiologically in certain limited types of cases (such as the temporary relief of nausea and pain), but if it does, it does so on a physiological basis (such as counterirritation or reflexes), not on the basis of its Taoist premises. In other words, putting a needle in a certain point in the body will likely have an effect—perhaps relieving pain somewhere else—causing a sense of numbness or tingling. However, the effects are not due to tapping into an invisible channel and modifying a mythical life force known as qi, which is rooted more in the psychic than in the physical realm.[40]

Spiritual Cautions

There are those who warn that pagan-based practices such as TCM cannot be separated from their occult roots, and that submitting oneself to such practices makes one vulnerable to the occult. However, this is probably also related to the spiritual maturity of the client and their uncompromising faith in God and His Word. Separation can and does occur. Christians are like Western medical practitioners and scientists who are atheists but still study God's creation—thereby discovering general revelation. They can separate a physical treatment in the natural realm, a false pagan interpretation from the treatment and a practitioner's false beliefs from the Word of God in order to receive treatments without leaving themselves vulnerable to demonic forces. However, we recommend that you pray before, during and after the treatment and that you not submit to any procedure that bypasses your conscious state of mind.

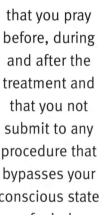

> We recommend that you pray before, during and after the treatment and that you not submit to any procedure that bypasses your conscious state of mind.

The distinction we are drawing is similar to the practice of martial arts. There is nothing wrong with the physical exercises that they are employing, and in a general sense, the same holds true for yoga exercises. However, if one has to bow to a divine master, then you'd better leave. Or if you have to pay homage to their beliefs, then you should not participate. On another note, it should not surprise us that various cultures of the world have discovered the herbs that God created are beneficial to our health. However, what must be discarded are their explanations that clearly contradict God's Word and natural law.

FINAL THOUGHTS

A scientist would understand acupuncture to be nothing more than some kind of interference with the electrochemical system of our bodies. It is likely affecting the transmission of neurotransmitters of which dopamine is the most likely. If you feel led to try acupuncture, we recommend that you seek treatment within the context of scientific medicine. For most believers, TCM should be avoided when the explanation for its effects are given in terms of energy or qi. Qigong clearly taps into the realm of the spiritual, especially with respect to qigong masters and emitted qi. Make no mistake about it, the occult works, but it is an abomination to God and will lead to spiritual bondage.

Modern TCM practitioners dismiss these objections, saying that the problem is with Western man's biomedical model of thinking, which interferes with man's ability to understand the validity of these ancient Chinese concepts. But if the Christian has to discard Scripture, natural law and the ability to reason, then he or she has nothing left but an empty mind, which becomes a vacuum for any and every idea that comes his or her way.

> The prudent sees the evil and hides himself, but the naive go on, and are punished for it (Prov. 22:3).

What is often overlooked in our Western world is the role that Satan and his demons can play within the realm of medicine and diseases. The Early Church seemed to have a different understanding of the reality of the spiritual world. Tertullian was a learned and skilled rhetorician in Carthage in northern Africa. He wrote his *Apology* for Christianity about A.D. 200. In this work he included an extended discussion of demons. The following is an excerpt from his writings:

> We are instructed, moreover, by our sacred books how from certain angels, who fell of their own free will, there sprang a more wicked demon brood, condemned of God along with the authors of their race, and their chief [Satan]. It will for the present be enough, however, that some account is given of their work. Their great business is the ruin of mankind. So from the very first, spiritual wickedness sought our destruction. They inflict, accordingly upon our bodies diseases and other grievous calamities, while by violent assaults they hurry the soul into sudden and extraordinary excesses. . . . Very kind to, no doubt, they are in regard to the healing of diseases. For, first of all, they make you ill; then to get a miracle out of it, they command the application of remedies either altogether new, or contrary to those in use, and straightway withdrawing hurtful influence they are supposed to have wrought a cure.[41]

Tertullian identified perhaps the greatest danger in spiritually counterfeit health paradigms. The appearance of success from a deceptive standpoint is to convince the user that the philosophy upon which the practice is based is true. Consider the scenario of Moses and pharaoh's magicians who at first were able to duplicate every one of Moses' miracles. But their power was not of God. As one preacher put it: At halftime, the score was tied. As we will put it: Don't base your conclusions merely upon the appearance of success.

CHAPTER FIFTEEN

IRIDOLOGY AND REFLEXOLOGY

IRIDOLOGY

Iridology is "the study of the iris, particularly of its color, markings, changes, etc., as associated with disease."[1] According to the theory of iridology (also known as iris examination), various organs are mapped onto the iris (the colored portion of the eye) in a clock-face pattern with 12 sectors. However, the claims of iridologists extend beyond the detection of physical disease. John Morley from the Iridology Research Institute says the eye is "where the nervous system comes to the surface and the iris reflects, via the nervous system, all parts of the body, and hence the mind and spirit, too."[2]

Evaluating Through the Grid of History

While playing in the woods as an 11-year-old Hungarian boy, Ignatz von Peczely was attacked by a mother owl. In an attempt to escape, Ignatz broke the owl's leg. Upon doing so, he noticed a black line appear in the iris of the owl. Years later, while training in Vienna as a natural practitioner and homeopath, von Peczely noticed a defect in the iris of a patient with a broken leg. Recalling his boyhood experience, he theorized that all disease was manifested in the iris of the eye.[3]

Von Peczely first published his ideas in 1864, then again in 1880 in *Discoveries in the Field of Natural Science in Medicine*. His concepts were accepted among many naturopaths and brought to the United States in 1904 by Dr. Henry Lahn, who that year published *Iridology: The Diagnosis from the Eye*.[4]

Subsequent American books on iridology include Bernard Jensen's *The Science and Practice of Iridology* (Red Wheel/Weiser, 1952), its sequel, *Iridology: Science and Practice in the Healing Arts* (Bernard Jensen, Intl., 1982) and Theodore Kriege's *Fundamental Basis of Iris Diagnosis* (Fowler, 1975).

Evaluating Through the Grid of Faith

We were unable to discover von Peczely's religious beliefs. However, the concept of an organ serving as a microcosm of the entire human body (macrocosm) comes from Taoism (see chapter 14). It actually first surfaced in the West in the sixteenth century through Paracelsus. A Swiss alchemist and physician, Paracelsus (A.D. 1493-1541) became disenchanted with Western medicine, traveled east—where he learned alternative medical philosophies—and then returned to Salzburg to practice his newfound ideology. He was rejected by a majority of the medical community.[5]

Some Christians in an attempt to find biblical support for iridology have cited Jesus' words from Matthew 6:22-24. However, we feel that the context of this passage does not support iridology.

> The lamp of the body is the eye; if therefore your eye is clear, your whole body will be full of light. But if your eye is bad, your whole body will be full of darkness. If therefore the light that is in you is darkness, how great is the darkness! No one can serve two masters; for either he will hate the one and love the other, or he will hold to one and despise the other. You cannot serve God and mammon.

The context is dealing with what you treasure and whom you trust. Seeking treasures on Earth through misplaced trust is the basis for anxiety.

Notice from the text that the information is not being read out through the eye; rather, the eye is the source of that which enters the body. It is the lamp that illuminates, not the screen that reports. Ancient tradition viewed the eyes as the windows through which light entered the body. If the eyes were in good condition, the whole body would receive the benefits that light bestows. If in bad condition, the whole body would plunge into darkness, which breeds disease. Jesus was not referring to light emitting from the sun. He was talking about spiritual illumination of which He is the light source. Our eyes of faith must be one, or else we will be double minded, and a double-minded person is unstable in all his or her ways (see Jas. 1:8). Therefore, the answer is to:

> Seek first His kingdom and His righteousness; and all these things shall be added to you (Matt. 6:33).

Evaluating Through the Wholistic Grid

An iridologist normally begins his or her assessment by taking a detailed history of the patient's symptoms. Then the eyes are examined with particular attention given to the iris. Equipment varies from a flashlight and magnifying glass to expensive optical and photographic technology. Pictures of the eye are projected onto a screen where both patient and practitioner can view them. The practitioner looks for irregularities in the fibrous tissue that makes up the iris and records his findings. Positive findings are correlated with an iridology chart. Then a diagnosis is rendered.

> We simply cannot treat the whole person as though it is unrelated to what he or she believes in the mind.

Iridologists claim that the right iris reflects the organs on the right side of the body, and the left iris reflects organs on the left side. They also say that these nerve signals come in through the optic nerve (the nerve directly attached to the back of the eyeball that carries visual images from the retina to the brain for interpretation).

One dimension overlooked in iridology and reflexology is the role of the mind. For example, data obtained from sight is sent to the brain but interpreted by how the mind has been programmed. The mind is tied to the physical body. Therefore, we simply cannot treat the whole person as though it is unrelated to what he or she believes in the mind. The eye is merely the means by which we see the world around us.

Evaluating Through the Grid of Science

It is standard practice in scientific medicine to examine the eye for disease. Diseases of the eye are numerous. For example, the whites of the eyes can become infected (pink eye). Dark material (cataracts) can form in the vitreous humor (the clear liquid) and obstruct vision. The retina can tear off (detach) from the lining inside of the eye.

In addition to eye disease, this organ is routinely examined for signs of disease that is elsewhere in the body. One of the reasons for this is that the retina is the only place on an external exam where a physician can transparently see blood vessels. For example, diabetes and high blood pressure may manifest themselves through changes in these delicate blood vessels. In addition, the whites of the eyes can become yellowed (jaundiced) when there are increased levels of bilirubin in the blood (e.g., liver disease, such as hepatitis) or discolored through an accumulation of toxins, such as in advanced kidney disease. However, the consensus in Western medicine is that the iris is a poor indicator of specific systemic disease.

Flawed Anatomical Concepts in Iridology Theory. While we don't want to establish bias before looking at clinical trials, we can tell that iridology is probably going to have serious problems with natural law simply because there are three major anatomical flaws in iridology theory.[6]

1. There is no neurological connection between the iris and the optic nerve.
2. The optic nerve is an afferent nerve. It's like a one-way street that sends information (i.e., pictures of what the eye sees) away from the eye to the brain. It does not bring any messages back to it. This has been well established through research.
3. Nearly all of the nerves in the body cross over to the other side of the spinal cord. Thus, if iridology were true, one should find organs from the right side of the body to be manifested in the left iris, not the right, as claimed by iridologists.

Despite these major, obvious flaws in theory, some iridologists claim that it is the single most important diagnostic tool ever:

We must realize that iridology represents a law of nature that cannot be changed. I believe that it is just as immutable and unchangeable as any of the laws that govern the universe.[7]

But a more objective review of its validity tends to suggest otherwise.

Research. One of iridology's earliest known challenges occurred around 1900. A renowned iridologist and naturopath by the name of Dr. Felke was put on trial before a jury. He was presented with 20 patients with serious diseases who were known to the jury but not to him. He was then asked to examine the eyes of each of the patients and render a diagnosis. He failed to properly diagnose the serious illness in all 20 cases.[8]

In a similar, but more recent challenge, Dr. Klaeser was tested to determine if he could properly diagnose patients with advanced ailments and mutilations. These ailments were so severe that they were obvious even to medical laymen. After failing at eight successive attempts, the experiment was discontinued. One patient with an amputated leg was said to have only "marked congestion of the spinal cord."[9]

In a study of 762 patients, 60 of whom were army veterans and many with amputations, a noniridologist physician examined their irises and then compared the findings to an iridology chart. Only 18 of the patients (2.7 percent) had a sign in an area of the chart that was associated with the obviously diseased organ. Furthermore, over 50 percent had disease signs in areas of the chart that were associated with normal organs.

Another report indicated that iridology was ineffective in diagnosing patients with an inflamed gallbladder containing gallstones. Stereo color slides were made of the right eye of 39 patients with this disease and of the right eye of 39 control subjects of the same sex and age. The slides were presented in random order to five leading iridologists without supplementary information. Overall, the iridologists were able to correctly identify the disease in slightly more than 50 percent of the cases (50 percent being the baseline for random chance).[10]

Similarly, a British study involving the comparison of iris photographs between normal subjects and those with disease affirmed that iridology was unable to aid in the diagnosis of ulcerative colitis, asthma, coronary heart disease and psoriasis. Each of these illnesses represents a severe form of disease of the particular system in question (i.e., intestines, lungs, heart and skin).[11]

In conjunction with the University of California, a study was conducted at the Veterans Administration Hospital in which photographs of the irises of patients were presented to three iridologists to see if they were able to accurately diagnose kidney disease by looking at the eye. The photographs were taken with a high quality Nikkor lens and ring flash. All parameters of the study were presented to and approved of by the iridologists in advance. The practitioners were presented with 143 patients, 95 of whom had no kidney disease (as defined by a serum creatinine of below 1.2 mg/dL), 24 of which had mild-to-moderate kidney disease (serum creatinine of 1.6-4.9) and 24 had severe kidney disease (serum creatinine of 6.3-16.0). Most of the latter group required routine dialysis because their kidneys were in complete failure. The findings of the study are summarized in the table below.[12]

	% of Patients with Disease		**% of Patients Without Disease**		
Iridologist	**True Positive (Sensitivity)**	**False Negative**	**True Negative (Specificity)**	**False Positive**	**P**
A	57	43	57	43	.07
B	37	63	44	56	.27
C	88	12	12	88	.42

Two of the iridologists were chiropractors and one was a non-health-care professional who had been apprenticed by one of the iridologists and practiced for several years. Iridologist A was a world-renowned expert and author of the most-popular text in iridology. He was the most accurate of the three, correctly identifying patients with kidney disease 57 percent of the time. However, he incorrectly diagnosed 57 percent of the normal patients to have kidney disease as well. In other words, he identified changes in the iris that revealed kidney disease in over half of the patients when there was no kidney disease. Even worse was iridologist B, who only identified 37 percent of the kidney disease patients and misdiagnosed 44 percent of the normal patients to have kidney disease. At first, iridologist C appeared to be more accurate, properly identifying 88 percent of the kidney disease patients. However, he also said 88 percent of the normal people had kidney disease. If one were to flip a coin as to the presence of kidney disease in each patient, there would be a 50 percent chance of making a correct diagnosis. Thus, despite the optimal technology and over 40 years of iridology experience, even the best iridologist performed no better than random guessing.

The authors of this research paper did a very interesting thing: They looked at the predictive value of iridology as a screening tool. Since kidney disease occurs in about two percent of the general population, about 20 people out of 1,000 in the general population will have it and 980 will not. The most accurate iridologist was iridologist A. If he were presented with 1,000 people out of the general population, he would properly identify 11 out of the 20 with kidney disease (57 percent times 20). However, he would tell 421 (57 percent times 980) that they had kidney disease when they really did not (i.e., false positives). Since the predictive value of a test is defined as the true positives (11), divided by the sum of the true positives, plus the false positives (11+421=432), the probability that it would be accurate in any given patient is only two and a half percent (11/432=2.5)!

Other Thoughts. Subsequent research has proven that breaking an owl's leg leaves no such mark in the iris.[13] Lacking scientific validation, most physicians in the West rejected (and continue to reject) the idea that the iris is neurologically connected to, and able to reflect changes in, every tissue in the body.[14] Some believe that what the young Dr. von Peczely saw was merely the visual effect produced by the black inner lining of the unique upper lid when the owl opens the eye. And so it seems clear by any objective analysis that iridology is a clinically worthless diagnostic tool.

Nevertheless, there are reports of individuals using it who are said to be extremely accurate. This can often be explained by the fact that iridologists are often vague in their description of an individual's disease. Furthermore, most patients who are suffering from a disease can have a diagnosis rendered merely on the basis of a thorough medical history. However, when the iridologist's accuracy tends to be much greater than that which has been established by objective testing—such as demonstrated in the University of California study or as explained by other factors as just mentioned in this paragraph—one must consider the possibility of psychic/occult involvement.

Evaluating Through the Grid of Spiritual Discernment

When asked whether or not a psychic ability was involved in iris diagnosis, one iridologist responded:

> Intuitive skills do come into play here, and whether we want to call this "psychic ability" or not . . . remains to be defined.[15]

Another author is quoted as saying that "many . . . practitioners use eye-diagnosis mediumistically," which would explain why someone with little or no medical training could be adept at diagnosing illness.[16]

Iridology should be rejected as a legitimate scientific diagnostic aid based on several reasons.

1. The initial premise is false. Subsequent research has proven that breaking an owl's leg leaves no distinguishing mark in the iris.

2. It is based upon faulty anatomical concepts.

3. There is substantial disagreement even among iridologists as to iris interpretation. Currently, there are at least 19 different iridology charts, all differing with one another enough that a diagnosis from one chart could conflict with one rendered from another chart.

4. Every known published objective report of an iridologist's ability to diagnose disease by examination of the iris has demonstrated an ability that is no better than random guessing.

5. When an iridologist is reported to have amazing accuracy, there is the possibility that it may not be through his or her scientific merits of iridology, but rather through his or her use of a mediumistic aid in diagnosis.

REFLEXOLOGY

Reflexology is "the science or study of reflexes."[17] It's also known as acupressure of the foot. Several years ago, a close acquaintance approached me (Michael) and enthusiastically related that he was recently cured of a problem with his pancreas. Since I knew that diseases of the pancreas tend to be anything but minor—and since I had known him well for years and was under the impression that he was in the best of health—I was surprised by his pronouncement. "That's exciting," I responded. "But I was not aware that you had a problem with your pancreas." He then went on to explain that he had visited a local reflexologist who, upon examining his feet, reported to him that he had a diseased pancreas. The reflexologist assured him that the condition was treatable by massage to the related area on his foot. Once the massage was completed, the reflexologist pronounced him "cured" of his pancreatic troubles.

If reflexology is true to its claims, it is awesome. We have the ability to diagnose and treat the whole body by just feeling and rubbing the feet. It would be easy to learn (anyone could do it) and, therefore, inexpensive (you wouldn't have to pay for a doctor's education, hospitalization, surgery, lab tests, etc.). Best of all, it is a pleasant experience. Who doesn't like a foot massage?

Evaluating Through the Grid of History

Reflexology evolved out of an earlier European system known as zone therapy and was introduced to America by William Fitzgerald, M.D., a Connecticut laryngologist. "Dr. Fitzgerald discovered he could induce numbness and alleviate certain symptoms in the body by applying finger pressure to specific points on the hands and mouth."[18] Using Fitzgerald's work as a basis, physiologist Eunice Ingham (Mrs. Fred Stopfel) mapped the body's organs onto the feet and developed techniques that she claimed could treat dysfunction of any of those organs. She called it reflexology and made it popular in America by writing the book *Stories the Feet Can Tell* (Ingham Publishing, Inc., 1932).

Evaluating Through the Grid of Faith

Like iridology, reflexology is rooted in Chinese Taoism, which contains the ancient concept of microcosm and macrocosm. This is the idea that all organs of the human body (the macrocosm) can be seen in (i.e., mapped out on) any single organ (the microcosm). Therefore, disease of any organ can be diagnosed and even treated at that single microcosm organ (in this case, the foot).[19] As explained below, the alternative form, often referred to as reflexotherapy, takes a purely mechanistic approach.

Evaluating Through the Wholistic Grid

Reflexology is "based on the proposition that the life force operates through ten channels as yet undiscovered by physiologists or neurologists."[20] These channels begin or end in the toes. Each channel relates to a zone of the body and the organs within that zone. In foot reflexology, the feet are examined for blocked energy channels, as evidenced by crystalline deposits or lumps under the skin. These are sought for and then treated with massage until they dissolve, which indicates that the energy channel and its related zone and organs are now free of disease.[21]

Reflexotherapy is the treatment by irritation of any area of the body distant from the lesion. Although it sounds very similar to reflexology, and its name is often used interchangeably, reflexotherapy is based upon an entirely different premise. Reflexotherapy (also referred to in Europe by some as neural therapy or neuroreflexotherapy) hypothesizes that there are points, or areas, all over the body that can be stimulated to reflexively influence another point, area or organ of the body. In this latter approach, the effects are believed to be mediated through nerves rather than through energy meridians and qi.

To illustrate this concept, let's look at a couple of examples that may be familiar to you. When the gallbladder becomes diseased, it can cause pain in the right shoulder area because the gallbladder and right shoulder share a related nerve supply. Likewise, someone suffering from a heart attack may experience pain in the left side of the neck or jaw, or in the left arm. But these examples involve purely sensory (afferent) reflexes. In other words, a problem in an organ (such as injury to the heart muscle during a heart attack) causes nerve impulses to be transmitted back to the spinal cord. There it interacts with nearby or related sensory nerves coming from another part of the body (e.g., the neck, jaw, left arm) so that the brain perceives that those areas are experiencing injury as well (when in fact they are perfectly fine). I (Neil) have struggled with kidney stones that often feel like a severe backache. Sometimes the pain seems to be in the groin, which is not diseased.

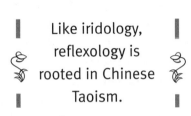

Like iridology, reflexology is rooted in Chinese Taoism.

Osteopathy and chiropractic take this concept one step further. As we discussed in chapters 11 and 12, osteopathy and chiropractic both contend that neurological pathways play a role in the proper function of organs. Restrictions in vertebral segments of the spine are believed to cause dysfunction in nerves, which are related to the vertebral levels of the spinal cord. These disruptions in nerve function lead to problems in the organs of innervation. Still and Palmer proposed and developed techniques for spinal manipulation to correct dysfunctional spinal vertebrae, believing that this would improve nerve function and thereby benefit the organs that were being served by those nerves. In other words, by correcting spinal problems, manipulation positively affects related organs by removing hindrances to the proper function of nerves (i.e., a passive affect).

Reflexotherapy takes neurological reflexes even one step further. It proposes that stimulation of sensory nerves on the surface of the body will go back to the spinal cord (no controversy at this point) and interact with nearby or related motor (efferent) nerves in order to effect a change in another organ (this is where the debate occurs). A simplified example of this is the familiar knee-jerk reflex. When your knee is tapped just below the kneecap with a reflex hammer, stretch receptors (i.e., sensory nerves) in the tendon are activated, sending a message up a nerve to the spinal cord. There the message instantly stimulates a motor nerve that innervates (supplies electrical stimuli to) the quadriceps muscle, causing it to contract, thus resulting in the knee jerk. At the same time, the sensory impulse is also transmitted up the spinal cord to the brain where it processes the information so that the individual feels and realizes that they have just been tapped below the knee.

To summarize the above process, surface stimulation of a sensory nerve triggered impulses in the motor nerve of another organ (the quadriceps muscle) to effect a change (contraction). But reflexotherapy asserts that surface stimulation can produce—through triggering motor nerve impulses—beneficial effects to related organs on a much grander scale than just triggering muscle contraction.

One of the proponents of this concept was Frank Chapman, an early-twentieth-century osteopath, who trained under A.T. Still. Chapman claimed that through the effects of neurological reflexes (which became known as Chapman's reflexes), one could both diagnose and treat disease from the body surface. For example, he taught that an infection of the middle ear (otitis media) causes a BB-sized tender nodule on the upper edge of the clavicle, near the first rib, and that stimulating this point would reflexively effect beneficial changes in the middle ear through alterations in not only nerve supply, but also blood and lymph flow. (Chapman also embraced naturopathic concepts, such as autointoxication.)[22]

Electro acupuncture, which is gaining increasing popularity in Europe and North America, is a modern variation of reflexotherapy. Electro acupuncture uses an instrument to electrically stimulate specific points to reflexively affect other areas or organs. While use of the term "acupuncture" might lead one to assume that the practice has a basis in traditional Chinese medicine, its practitioners usually explain that it works through neurological reflexes (like reflexotherapy), not on the TCM basis of manipulating a life force qi along invisible meridians.

Unfortunately, the terms "reflexology" and "reflexotherapy" are often used interchangeably, so it can be difficult at first glance to know whether the practice is claiming to be based upon Taoist energy meridians and qi or upon neurological principles. However, although the two methods are basing their theories on two very different mechanisms, in some respects they are addressing essentially the same questions, using similar methods of diagnosis and treatment.

Evaluating Through the Grid of Science

With regard to diagnosis, both reflexology and reflexotherapy contend that one can diagnose organ problems by palpitation (touching the body with the hands to feel for abnormalities). In reflexology, the locations of irregularities (such as nodules) are compared to a standard reflexology chart, which maps all of the body's organs onto the foot according to the positions of their respective meridians. In reflexotherapy, the locations of irregularities are compared to charts that are believed to represent neurological reflexes or pathways. Whichever organ correlates with that location is believed to be diseased.

To test this idea, we looked for studies in which reflexologists were asked to examine the feet of individuals with known diseases and render the patient's diagnosis without knowing his or her medical history. We only found one study, and while it had some design flaws, it concluded that reflexologists were very inaccurate in diagnosing disease (this is despite the fact that one of the authors was a 10-year veteran reflexologist).[23] (See table B-3 for further details on this study.)

In addition, to evaluate the effectiveness of reflexology and reflexotherapy in treating disease, we looked for studies of individuals with known diseases in which either approach was used as treatment. Of course, the best studies are those that are controlled in such a way that the patient is not aware of whether they are truly receiving reflexology. In particular, those studies in which the feet are massaged but care is taken to avoid stimulating the zones corresponding to the diseased organs would seem optimal, because this would help to differentiate whether or not any beneficial effects were due to reflexology/reflexotherapy or merely to 30 minutes of relaxing physical touch. (See table B-4 for a summarized list of these studies.)

From a scientific standpoint, there is disagreement among researchers as to whether or not reflexology or reflexotherapy really work. As with iridology, the central premise of microcosm should be easy to test—the organs of the body can be mapped out on the surface of the body and disease can be diagnosed by feeling for irregularities in that surface. However, there should be more studies in which reflexologists are challenged in a blinded fashion to diagnose patients who may or may not have severe disease, as confirmed by other accepted methods. If reflexology were a legitimate science, the reflexologist should be able to accurately diagnose the illness by only examining the foot, ear, hand or whatever is being claimed as the microcosm organ.

 Without critically evaluating a philosophy's precepts with the five grids described in this book, we can become spiritually desensitized.

The second concept—that one can treat disease in distant organs through applying pressure to points or zones on the skin—is even less proven. In summarizing the research presented in table B-4, the evidence is less than overwhelming. Despite the nearly 100-year presence of reflexology in America, almost nothing has been published in American or English medical journals, and controlled studies are sorely lacking, which leaves an inquirer who is looking for objective, reliable proof quite empty-handed.

Evaluating Through the Grid of Spiritual Discernment

We do not see good evidence that these practices truly accomplish what they claim—that disease can be diagnosed and treated through examination and pressure to the skin surface. In fact, other than the obvious benefit of a relaxing foot rub, the evidence seems to point the other way. Nevertheless, the practices appear to be physically harmless, so long as the patient does not have a diagnosis that is being missed and for which more effective treatment is available.

As noted above, the concept of microcosm is rooted in Taoism, a pagan religion with numerous precepts contrary to Christianity. However, to our knowledge, the practices of reflexology and reflexotherapy do not inherently impinge upon the spiritual realm unless it affects our beliefs. In that regard, we see potential spiritual danger from two avenues:

1. If the practitioner is involved in occult or psychic activities. We should be cautious concerning who puts their hands on us. Touch is an important part of intimate relationships, and it has a lot to do with trust. We are urged by the mercies of God to submit our bodies

to Him (see Rom. 12:1) but not to any other people unless we are sure that we can trust them.

2. If the medical practice of reflexology is accepted (or any other medical philosophy rooted in paganism). Without critically evaluating a philosophy's precepts with the five grids described in this book, we can become spiritually desensitized, causing us to become less discerning in other matters as well (this should be especially apparent if we find ourselves becoming defensive about the employment of a practice incompatible with biblical faith). Indeed, this is how various forms of New Age medicine can act as a "gateway drug" to deeper spiritual deception and bondage.

CHAPTER SIXTEEN

APPLIED KINESIOLOGY (AK)

EVALUATING THROUGH THE GRID OF HISTORY

Applied kinesiology (AK) is an approach to diagnosing and treating illness that was founded by George Goodheart, Jr., a Michigan chiropractor.[1] Upon examining a young male patient with chronic shoulder pain in 1964, Dr. Goodheart noticed that his client's scapula muscles were weak and that they contained multiple, painful nodules at their insertions to the rib cage. Since the problem had failed to respond to conventional chiropractic manipulation, Dr. Goodheart tried something different. He applied heavy, rotary pressure to the nodules. "To the doctor's surprise and the patient's delight, there was an immediate disappearance of the shoulder pain and complete normalization of serratus anterior function, including full strength to muscle testing. This incident was the starting point for investigation into the significance of muscle weakness."[2]

Applied kinesiology has gained immense popularity, particularly among chiropractors. More than one out of every three chiropractors in the U.S. utilize it. Even higher use is reported among chiropractors in other countries. It has also gained many converts among dentists, as well as some physicians.[3] Accordingly, Goodheart has organized its practitioners, forming the International College of Applied Kinesiology (ICAK), which holds conferences and publishes research on AK.

Evaluating Through the Grid of Faith

Some have claimed that Goodheart was psychic and developed his charts through occult methods.[4] In a personal letter to me (Michael), Goodheart flatly denied this, stating that such assertions were baseless and contrary to his Roman Catholic faith.[5] While we certainly accept this, we often seem to find AK (or at least variations on the theme) being used in settings and ways that are of a spiritually (and professionally) questionable nature. Perhaps Goodheart may not have intended such occultlike similarities, but in looking at where he got some of his ideas, it should not be surprising.

Evaluating Through the Wholistic Grid

After his initial discovery, Goodheart studied various writings on the concepts of muscle weakness and their relationship to reflexes. The next year, he added ideas developed by osteopath Frank Chapman (see chapters 14 and 15) who believed that diseased organs manifested themselves through nerve reflexes with irregularities on the skin that could be felt as tender nodules. They contended that these nodules could be stimulated and, through what became known as Chapman's reflexes, result in improved function of the related organs and in the flow of body fluids. Goodheart combined this idea with his muscle testing, hypothesizing that each organ that was diseased would not only produce "trigger points" but also be associated with a weak muscle.[6]

> Applied kinesiology has gained immense popularity, particularly among chiropractors.

Later, Goodheart added another theory known as neurovascular dynamics (NVD) that was developed in the 1930s by chiropractor Terrence Bennett. Bennett believed that adults still had remnants of the embryological pulse (i.e., the circulatory system of the very early embryo in the mother's womb). He claimed that pulse centers could be activated by touching them, which would in turn stimulate blood supply to specific areas of the body.

Goodheart also became familiar with the work of William G. Sutherland, D.O., an osteopath who discovered the supposed movement of cranial (skull) bones and their relationship to the flow of cerebrospinal fluid (CSF). Finally, after reading Felix Mann, M.D.'s book on acupuncture, *The Ancient Chinese Art of Healing*, Goodheart embraced the concept that acupressure and acupuncture points were associated with internal organs, and that internal organ function could be affected by stimulation of these specific points. Again, Goodheart combined this idea with his theory of muscle weakness being associated with internal organ disease. TCM terminology and meridian concepts are often acknowledged in AK writings.

In 1972, Goodheart added the vertebral challenge technique developed by Lewis Truscott, D.C., in which slight pressure is applied to a vertebral segment (particularly in the neck) and the leg lengths are checked. According to Truscott, if there is a subluxation (malposition) at the vertebra that is pressed, it will show up as a change in leg length. Goodheart modified Truscott's technique, claiming that when a subluxated vertebra is challenged, it will result in muscular weakness.

The next year, he added his own invention, therapy localization. With this technique, the doctor touches the patient at a reflex point and tests the muscle strength of its corresponding muscle. If the physician touching the point makes the muscle weaker or stronger, it indicates the need for treatment in the area.

According to the ICAK website, applied kinesiology is:

1. A diagnostic system using muscle testing to augment normal examination procedures.

2. A diagnostic tool that uses the neuromuscular system and other measurable parameters to aid in evaluating what is wrong and what to do for a patient.

3. An applied kinesiology examination depends upon knowledge of functional neurology, anatomy, physiology, biomechanics and biochemistry and is combined with standard physical examination procedures, laboratory findings, X rays and history taking.

4. The different procedures developed by Dr. Goodheart and others are derived from many disciplines including chiropractic, osteopathy, medicine, dentistry, acupuncture, biochemistry, etc. and are currently being used by doctors of chiropractic, osteopathy, homeopathy, dentistry and medicine.

5. An expanding body of knowledge that covers in depth the structural and chemical imbalances that are at the base of most patient's problems.

6. Based on chiropractic principles and requires manual manipulation of the spine, extremities and cranial bones as the structural basis of its procedures.[7]

In summary, applied kinesiology is the amalgamation of several different theories. First, weak or atonic muscles can be strengthened by treating their attachments with pressure. Second, specific reflex points in the body are associated with diseased organs (Chapman—neurolymphatic reflexes). Third, touching specific points can stimulate blood flow to specific areas (Bennett—NVD). Fourth, cerebrospinal fluid movement is related to cranial bone motion and is important for optimum health (Sutherland—cranial). Fifth, acupuncture and acupressure points can be stimulated with pressure to affect internal organs (Mann—TCM). Sixth, subluxated vertebrae, when challenged, will manifest with associated muscle weakness (Truscott). Finally, reflex points, when challenged, will indicate a problem if muscle strength decreases or increases.

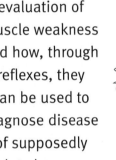

> Applied kinesiology is the evaluation of muscle weakness and how, through reflexes, they can be used to diagnose disease of supposedly related organs.

If you are confused, don't feel bad. This complicated set of ideas is difficult to coalesce into a clear, understandable, succinct statement. In reality, AK is the evaluation of muscle weakness and how, through reflexes, they can be used to diagnose disease of supposedly related organs. Psychosomatic illnesses are not addressed nor is the faith foundation of the practitioner or client.

EVALUATING THROUGH THE GRID OF SCIENCE

Most articles that support AK are found in the *AK Review* and in a compilation of essays by AK practitioners, entitled the *Collected Papers of the ICAK*. Both are publications of the International College of Applied Kinesiology (ICAK). Klinkoski and Leboeuf conducted a review of 50 papers published by the ICAK between 1981 and 1987, 20 of which were classified as "research papers." They reported that none of the selected ICAK papers met all seven of the basic criteria essential to research methodology.[8]

One book claims that "a competent AK practitioner may, indeed, perform vital health services unmatched in the healing arts" and that AK testing will eventually be proven "extremely accurate" if not "infallible."[9] But at least the mainstream scientific literature seems to point to the contrary: "Many of the peer-reviewed papers that have been published regarding AK methodology have been either negative or inconclusive in their results."[10]

In papers that examined some of the premises underlying applied kinesiology, Dr. Haas found that muscle strength was not a valid indicator of vertebral "subluxation."[11] He also concluded that the use of leg-length discrepancy in Truscott's vertebral challenge method was a "diagnostic illusion" and "not . . . viable for identifying vertebrae for adjustment."[12] In other words, according to Haas, the vertebral challenge premise proposed by Truscott doesn't work.

Lawson and Calderon challenged three experienced applied kinesiologists to see if they could independently agree on their estimation of muscle strength. The bottom line: Half the time they agreed with one another and half the time they did not.[13] Kenney found that practitioners tended to not only disagree with one another, but also with a muscle testing machine (dynamometer) and the laboratory.[14]

We could find only one article in the National Library of Medicine that seemed to support AK methodology, and that was an uncontrolled study done in Israel in which AK was used to screen patients for food allergies. They were then tested with conventional laboratory testing of those same foods. (See table B-5 for a summarized look at available mainstream AK studies.)

While it is certainly possible that the methodology being tested or being used by various AK practitioners would not have measured up to the standards of Dr. Goodheart and the International College of Applied Kinesiology (ICAK), these studies are all we have to go on. At the very least, it should raise questions as to either the legitimacy of AK theory or its accuracy in the hands of many practitioners.

EVALUATING THROUGH THE GRID OF SPIRITUAL DISCERNMENT

As mentioned earlier, some people have expressed concern that Goodheart had connections with the occult—an assertion he flatly denies. In his own words, "I am a Catholic by religion . . . and in my opinion a fellow Christian by devotion . . . My AK research activity and discoveries came from much hard work, much trial and error, many late nights, many problems and some successes. None of this effort came from psychic sources." He refers to such claims as a "monstrous distortion of fact."[15] Likewise, the ICAK website has this to say about what AK is not:

1. A simple yes or no, radionics or pendulum type of testing system.
2. Testing bottles in the hand or pills on the skin.
3. Testing or using mental telepathy.
4. Using crystals or magnets as treatment modalities.
5. Touch For Health or any of the other forms of evaluation using muscle testing as a simple yes or no answer system.
6. A simplistic, cookie-cutter approach to treatment.[16]

From reading the list, you can get an idea of the kind of criticism that has been leveled at AK practitioners. Despite Dr. Goodheart's intention that AK is kept purely in the realm of the physical, not everyone who uses muscle testing respects that wish. We have personally encountered numerous objectionable situations.

Recall in chapter 2 that the practitioner monitored muscle strength (or leg length or whatever) while asking the body to tell him the correct dose. This appears to be virtually no different than using a pendulum (radionics) to get a yes or no answer from the spirit realm. In their book on AK, Tom and Carole Valentine excitedly report on the "ongoing experimentation" by AK researchers who are using pendulums to "dowse" food and nutritional supplements (i.e., determine if they are good or bad for you).[17] Similarly, muscle testing has been used for psychic purposes.[18]

We have received reports that the muscle testing only works if the patient believes in it. Other testimony has indicated that when the spirit behind the muscle testing was prayed against or renounced, the approach did not work.[19] Still, others have reported that practitioners have claimed that they can make diagnoses and prescribe treatment over the telephone through muscle testing. And in an even stranger application, a midwestern herbalist is reported to use muscle testing by tracing his finger down a wall chart while his associate muscle tests the patient. When the patient tests weak, he stops his finger; wherever it is pointing is the organ that is diseased. Such obvious departures from rational and biblical thinking should be readily apparent to any Christian. However, every one of the situations just described involved people who believed in the approach and claimed to be Christian.

CONCLUSION

Some of the ideas upon which applied kinesiology are based seem to be consistent with known anatomy and physiology, and have some degree of time-tested validity (e.g., neurological reflexes). Other aspects of this theory seem to be truly unfounded. For example, the vertebral challenge theory by Truscott has little support scientifically. Three papers appear to prove it a fallacy.

Most important, there is substantial evidence that at least in the hands of certain practitioners, applied kinesiology may step over the line into occult involvement. This is not to say that all AK is that way. It is not. And certainly, much of what is labeled as AK is not what its founder intended. For these reasons, it is our recommendation that it either be avoided, or if used, used with caution and objective verification.

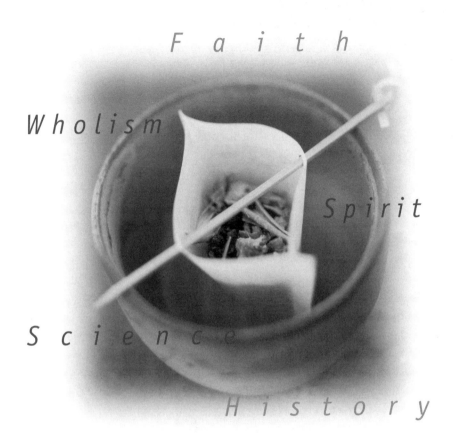

Faith

Wholism

Spirit

Science

History

PART 3

EVALUATING
ALTERNATIVE
THERAPIES

CHAPTER SEVENTEEN

DIET AND NUTRITION

The serpent said to the woman, "You surely shall not die! For God knows that in the day you eat from it your eyes will be opened, and you will be like God, knowing good and evil." When the woman saw that the tree was good for food, and that it was a delight to the eyes, and that the tree was desirable to make one wise, she took from its fruit and ate; and she gave also to her husband with her, and he ate.

GENESIS 3:4-6

EVALUATING THROUGH THE GRID OF HISTORY

Since the beginning of time, the world has not lacked for those who try to sell others on the miraculous qualities of special foods and diets, and many are their followers. Even Adam and Eve were deceived by such a claim. Today the market is glutted by diet books, each heralding a unique food or dietary approach that assures the reader of a long and blissful life—if ye will only take and eat.

Contrast that with my (Michael's) preparation for medicine. Even as a freshman chemistry student, I recall one of my college science professors concluding, "It does not matter what you eat. To a cell, glucose is glucose, no matter where it came from." Even though I was far less educated at the time, I sensed he was wrong. Is it possible that someone as knowledgeable as a college microbiologist didn't understand the importance of nutrition? Is there any truth to the old axiom You are [physically] what you eat?

Yes, he didn't understand, and there is truth to the old axiom. Many medical doctors have failed to recognize the value of a prudent diet, because the majority of physicians receive little or no coursework in nutrition while attending medical school. Nutrition has not been an essential part of the traditional Western medical paradigm. Allopathy, for instance, is a disease-oriented model that has relied heavily upon medication and other invasive treatments for its cures. Nutrition has not been perceived as part of the cure. This becomes embarrassingly obvious upon a patient's first introduction to hospital food. At a time when good nutrition is critical for recovery from illness or surgery, the sick are often provided with a dietary fare that does everything but hasten healing.

> **Nutrition has not been an essential part of the traditional Western medical paradigm.**

The poor nutritional value of hospital food had always puzzled me until I lectured to a group of registered dietitians (R.D.'s). They had invited me to speak on the use of nutrition to prevent and treat heart disease. After the lecture, several asked questions, since much of what I shared was new or contrary to what they were learning in school. When I asked why, they expressed frustration at the heavy influence of food manufacturing companies in their education, which they felt distorted their training. For example, they were shocked when I explained that butter, a product from nature and high in cholesterol, was actually better for heart patients than man-made margarine.[1] Most margarines contain hydrogenated vegetable oils and harmful trans fatty acids.[2] Similarly, they were also surprised to learn that eggs, although loaded with cholesterol, have never been shown to significantly raise blood levels for heart disease. One of the lowest cholesterol levels I have ever measured on a patient was 133—on a patient who ate 40 eggs per week! There appears to be no evidence that egg substitutes are healthier than God-given natural eggs.[3]

Registered dietitians are the experts in medicine who counsel patients on nutrition and design hospital menus for the sick. I have met and worked with many of them, all delightful, caring people. But all too often they, and physicians like myself whom they serve, are out of touch when it comes to being prepared to provide good counsel on nutrition. The void created by this absence has created a flood of "experts," each claiming to have the right nutritional plan for you.

EVALUATING THROUGH THE GRID OF FAITH

At first glance, one would think that diets and religion have nothing in common. However, many of the diets being proposed today are not based upon theories that fit the author's religious worldview. For example, some introduce their books with the assertion that our ancestors were primarily farmers. The belief that we were not designed for consuming meat forms the basis for their advocacy of vegetarianism. On the opposite end of the spectrum are those who claim that our lineage goes back to cavemen hunters and scavengers. They believe we are genetically programmed for a meat-based diet—high in protein and low in carbohydrates—the exact opposite of the vegetarian evangelists.[4]

Some diets were clearly birthed in formal religious systems. For example, a macrobiotic diet emphasizes eating in such a way as to be in harmony with the universe, its seasons and one's own body type.[5] This is characteristic of Eastern religious belief systems (see chapters 9 and 14) and finds some replication in Western diets that adjure followers to eat in accordance with their types—body, blood or otherwise.[6]

Far East faiths are not the only ones with dietary programs. Orthodox Jews adhere to the kosher diet, a modified version of the commandments given by God to the Hebrews in 1500 B.C.[7] In addition, throughout Christian history, there have been those who have looked to the Mosaic Law in an attempt to integrate faith, Scripture and diet in various ways. Most notable are the Seventh-day Adventists, who cite passages such as Leviticus 11 as the basis for their dietary convictions.[8] More recently, Dr. Rex Russell effectively pointed out the value of living in harmony with the dietary and hygiene laws of Moses.[9] While I (Michael) acknowledged the significance of these biblical commandments in *The Word on Health*, I attempted to explain them from the perspective of living under the new covenant of grace.[10]

Some believe that God's ideal diet is vegetarian, which He originally gave at creation (see Gen. 1:29). As we discussed in our section on naturopathy, this doctrinal position is not new, but was first seen in the West in the early 1800s at the birth of the natural hygiene movement.[11] Like the naturopathy that it spawned, many of those who adopt this perspective believe that all sickness is due to an accumulation of toxins and poor eating habits. Therefore, they propose that a change in diet will not only prevent disease but also cure it.

Since the purpose of this book is to evaluate medicine from a biblical worldview, does this claim line up with Scripture? While common sense and natural law tell you that diet is an important factor in the cause and prevention of illness, we must acknowledge that when it comes to blaming diet for all of our health problems or touting it as a cure for all of our diseases, there is scant scriptural evidence to support such an assertion. For example, in all likelihood, the great majority of the Jews were eating a diet that would be considered by most modern standards to be very healthy (only unrefined, naturally occurring organic foods, containing no chemical contaminants, a preponderance of whole grains, fruits and vegetables and only clean animal products). And yet, during His earthly ministry, Jesus was besieged by the sick in pursuit of healing (see Mark 6:53-56).

EVALUATING THROUGH THE GRID OF SCIENCE

We need to ask the question, Which diet has been scientifically proven to prevent and/or cure disease? The answer is none. Does that mean that there is no scientific basis for dietary recommendations? No, as we acknowledged, there is no doubt that a preponderance of evidence shows that sound nutrition is of tremendous value. First of all, some diets are particularly helpful in certain disease states. For example, individuals with lactose (milk and sugar) intolerance do much better when they avoid dairy products. Likewise, those with celiac disease cannot handle gluten-containing foods such as wheat, oats and barley. A physician friend who was critically ill with severe Crohn's disease saw his health dramatically improve when he went on a diet restrictive of specific carbohydrates.[12] However, these diets potentially benefit only select groups of people. You will have to do some personal research to determine if you are one of them.

Second, countless studies have validated the importance of dietary lifestyle in reducing the risk of our most common diseases. For example, heart disease has been associated with excess calories, excess intake of saturated or damaged fats (such as hydrogenated oils) and reduced intake of fruits and vegetables.[13] One study showed that the residents of the island of Crete had 98 percent less coronary artery disease than what is found in the United States![14] This was attributed mostly to the Crete residents' diet. Similarly, 35 percent of cancer, the second leading cause of death in the United States, has been linked to diet.[15]

This exceeds the influence of tobacco, which is believed to account for 30 percent of malignancies. If a person ate a prudent diet and did not smoke, he or she could theoretically reduce his or her risk of cancer by nearly two-thirds.

Finally, one would think that if sound nutrition proved to help prevent diseases such as cancer, then it would be helpful in treatment as well.[16] While we have both personally seen numerous examples of such cases, nevertheless, the scientific literature is very sparse regarding this contention. Dietary therapy is not an inherently allopathic concept, which is perhaps why such studies are so few and far between. While it seems logical that diet should play an important role in the treatment of disease, we cannot claim this on the basis of scientific studies.

Michael harmonized the scientific literature on diet and lifestyle with what the Bible says about these in *The Word on Health*. He summarized his results by giving 10 dietary suggestions:

1. Eat only what you need.
2. Get adequate exercise.
3. Eat "real" food; i.e., that which comes from nature.
4. Make plant foods central (fruits, vegetables, nuts, whole grains).
5. Drink plenty of pure water.
6. Prefer what the Bible defines as "clean" animal flesh.
7. Don't eat blood or improperly prepared meat.
8. Avoid the "hard" fat of animals.
9. Culture your dairy products.
10. Don't let diet take precedence over God or others.[17]

Rex Russell made it even simpler. He summarized biblical precepts regarding diet into three concepts.

1. Eat what God gave for food.
2. Don't alter His design.
3. Don't let any food or drink become your god.[18]

But it is this last concept that most dieters probably struggle with the most, since the most common reason for why someone pursues a dietary program is to lose weight. While each of today's fad diets tends to claim to be superior to its competitors, the fact is that not one has been scientifically proven to be so.[19]

This becomes obvious when you see the endless cycle that weight-loss hopefuls endure as they go from diet to diet, unsuccessfully trying the latest recommendation of a friend or the local bookstore. Other than the questionable claims upon which these diets are typically based, there is one major deficiency common to all of them—they don't come packaged with the ability to follow them.

There is no earthly diet that can be identified as God's diet. There are no certain foods that are in His program and certain foods that are out, since all natural foods have been created by God. Paul warned against:

Men who forbid marriage and advocate abstaining from foods, which God has created to be gratefully shared in by those who believe and know the truth. For everything created by God is good, and nothing is to be rejected, if it is received with gratitude; for it is sanctified by means of the word of God and prayer (1 Tim. 4:3-5).

> There are no certain foods that are in God's program and certain foods that are out, since all natural foods have been created by Him.

From the previous context, we know that Paul is giving an example of spiritual deception in the last days.

Our creator could have made just one food and given us that for every meal. Imagine if all we had to eat were brussels sprouts! He did supernaturally provide manna in the wilderness for 40 years, but the Israelites got so tired of it that they all wanted to go back to Egypt. God has made an incredible variety of food to suit every taste, culture and climate, and intends that we enjoy it. Our problem is really not for want of the right food, but the right spirit.

> For the kingdom of God is not eating and drinking, but righteousness and peace and joy in the Holy Spirit (Rom. 14:17).

EVALUATING THROUGH THE GRID OF SPIRITUAL DISCERNMENT

The apostle Paul said, "I can do all things through Christ who strengthens me" (Phil. 4:13, *NKJV*). Why is it then that the vast majority of people (including

Christians) who attempt to follow a dietary program do so unsuccessfully? The answer is actually quite simple and is found in the passage just quoted—they aren't doing it through Christ. We propose that there are three components to being able to have the strength of Christ "to do all things."

1. **Being in Christ.** Obviously, being in Christ is a prerequisite to enjoying the benefit of Him empowering your life. Jesus said, "Abide in me, and I in you. As the branch cannot bear fruit of itself, except it abide in the vine; no more can ye, except ye abide in me . . . for without me ye can do nothing" (John 15:4-5, *KJV*).

2. **Walking in the will of Christ.** "And this is the confidence that we have in him, that, if we ask any thing according to his will, he heareth us" (1 John 5:14, *KJV*). Is it God's will that you eat certain types or amounts of foods and avoid others? If so, then He makes His grace available to you. On the other hand, if it is not His will, you will have no more strength to follow that diet than someone who is not a Christian. Apart from Christ, we can do nothing (see John 15:5). Furthermore, God will not lead His children to follow a dietary plan whose precepts espouse faith in someone or something other than Himself.

3. **Depending upon the Spirit of Christ.** Most diets consist of two long lists and a law—eat the foods that are acceptable and don't eat those that are forbidden. With this law hanging over a person, it doesn't take long before the dieter is confronted with the same temptation that Eve experienced, and with the same results. There are two types of cravings for food. First, we crave certain foods because we have a biological need that needs fulfillment. If you are hungry, you should eat. The second craving is a lust for foods that taste good. Paul said, "Walk by the Spirit, and you *will not* carry out the desire of the flesh" (Gal. 5:16, emphasis added). The word "walk" in this verse is *peripateo*. It means to walk around an area with someone, like going for a walk in the park. It is a walk with God. As long as you live by faith in the power of the Holy Spirit, you will not carry out the desires of the flesh. Nobody living under the law can live up to the law, but if we live under the New Covenant of Grace, we can live a righteous life.

Diane Hampton, who is no stranger to dietary fads and failure, points out in her helpful book *The Diet Alternative* to follow Christ, not a diet. He will give you wisdom along with the grace (the power and desire to do God's will) you need.[20]

CONCLUSION

In reality, there is only one perfect food that guarantees an eternity of blissful health. Unfortunately, man is unable to access it. As a direct result of sin and its corrupting influence upon his nature, man was permanently barred from this life-giving food. The tree that produces it, once available in the garden of Eden, has since been transplanted to heaven where it abides, out of our reach. One day that will change; the perfect food will be accessible once again. But according to the God who created it, not everyone will have access to it. Instead, the right to eat of it will be given only to those who are alive in Christ. For He, the Bread of Life, who said that whoever came to Him would never hunger nor thirst again (see John 6:35), through the shedding of His own blood at Calvary (see Heb. 9:11-14), purchased the rights to that tree and, by His immeasurable graciousness, will freely give access privileges unto all who call upon His name.

> And he showed me a pure river of water of life, clear as crystal, proceeding out of the throne of God and of the Lamb. In the midst of the street of it, and on either side of the river, was there the tree of life, which bare twelve manner of fruits, and yielded her fruit every month: and the leaves of the tree were for the healing of the nations. Blessed are they that do his commandments, that they may have the right to the tree of life, and may enter in through the gates into the city (Rev. 22:1-2,14, *KJV*).

CHAPTER EIGHTEEN

HERBS, DRUGS AND SUPPLEMENTS

In addition to giving the perfect food, the tree of life also bore leaves for healing (see Rev. 22:2). When the prophet Ezekiel foretold of this great structure, he stated that its leaves were "for medicine" (Ezek. 47:12, *NKJV*). Scripture affirms what many secular historians have observed—herbs have been used as medicinal agents in virtually every culture since antiquity.

EVALUATING THROUGH THE GRIDS OF HISTORY, FAITH AND WHOLISM

Virtually all of the biblical references to the medicinal use of herbs involve their application to the surface of the body. When King Hezekiah got sick, he prayed and asked God for healing. God answered his prayer through the prophet Isaiah, who had a poultice of figs applied to the king's boil (see 2 Kings 20:7). Jeremiah made reference to a healing balm in Gilead (see Jer. 8:22; 46:11) but warned Israel that her wounds were incurable (see Jer. 30:12-13). Isaiah wrote, "The whole head is sick, and the whole heart faint. From the sole of the foot even unto the head there is no soundness in it; but wounds, and bruises, and putrifying sores: they have not been closed, neither bound up, neither mollified with ointment" (Isa. 1:5-6, *KJV*).

The Good Samaritan applied oil and wine to the wounds of the stranger who had been beaten (see Luke 10:34). James instructed sick Christians to call for the elders for prayer and to be anointed with oil (see Jas. 5:14). This anointing may refer to the application of topical medication. There are two Greek words in the New Testament used for "anoint." The first word is *creo*, which refers to anointing that is part of a ceremony or ritual. The second word is *aleipho*, which can refer to the application of an ointment for medicinal purposes. In James 5:14, the word *aleipho* is used.[1]

Nowhere in Scripture do we find Hebrews or Christians taking herbs or drugs orally. The closest that they appeared to come to it was in the form of a food when Paul encouraged Timothy to "drink no longer water, but use a little wine for thy stomach's sake and thine often infirmities" (1 Tim. 5:23, *KJV*). We now know that the juice of the grape contains antibacterial properties as well as antioxidants that can be helpful for gastrointestinal ailments. In addition, the Greek word *pharmakia*, from which we get our own word "pharmacy," literally means sorcery, witchcraft or remedies prepared with magic.[2]

Protect the Mind

These observations have led some to conclude that Christians should abstain from using all medicinal drugs, believing that their employment is tantamount to cooperating with the occult. While scripturally this argument may have some merit, there are probably other factors to consider when coming to a conclusion on this issue.

The pharmakia of those days was—as was much of medicine—heavily steeped in pagan worship and the occult. It is therefore inappropriate to indiscriminately apply the same definition to today's pharmaceutical industry. Nevertheless, there are three potential dangers in using drugs.

1. There is the possibility of becoming chemically addicted to prescription medications.
2. Some doctors prescribe with the hope that medication will solve all your problems. This may be a substitute for our hope in God.
3. Mind-altering drugs can induce a passive state of the mind, which can be spiritually dangerous.

Scripture specifically commands us to maintain control of our minds. Paul exhorted believers to "be not drunk with wine, wherein is excess; but be filled with the Spirit" (Eph. 5:18, *KJV*). In other words, do not allow yourself to come under the influence of alcohol (a drug) so that you allow it to affect your mind.

Perhaps this is one reason why alcoholic drinks have been referred to as spirits, since by them an individual can yield his mind to their influence. Instead, we have to assume responsibility for all our thoughts and make sure they are in obedience to Christ (see 2 Cor. 10:5). (We will discuss biblical "thought control" in greater depth in chapter 20.)

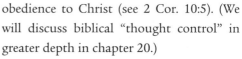

Just because a drug is legal does not mean that it cannot alter the mind.

What is not so obvious is the fact that just because a drug is legal does not mean that it cannot alter the mind and, therefore, make a person spiritually vulnerable. In fact, the expressed purpose of some drugs is to alter the mind, such as is the case with narcotics for pain and those used to treat psychosis, anxiety and depression. Therefore, it stands to reason that prudence should be especially exercised when it comes to using these classes of drugs, particularly when one considers the fact that these diagnoses often reflect underlying spiritual needs that should be addressed. Almost any drug can, if given in large enough doses, be toxic to the brain (and therefore the mind). I (Michael) recall a patient who began hallucinating when she was accidentally given an overdose of a local anesthetic. It took nearly one hour for the drug to clear enough that her mind could return to normal, during which time she was given supportive care and prayer for her protection.

Similarly, countless numbers of patients in operating rooms all across the globe surrender not only their bodies but also their minds to the surgeon's and anesthesiologist's complete control. Some have expressed concern that they see no difference spiritually between using a drug to induce general anesthesia and altering one's state of consciousness through hypnosis. When confronted with this objection, one of the early pioneers of general anesthesia thoughtfully pointed out that God himself set the precedent of general anesthesia when He compassionately put Adam into a deep sleep prior to conducting the world's premier surgery. Since God is not the one administering the anesthesia during surgery, it seems prudent before any surgical endeavor to call upon Him for protection of body, soul and spirit.

Know the Effects of Herbs

The oral use of herbs during biblical days was largely confined to pagan cultures whose religious belief systems were directly related to their practice of medicine. Only in the last several centuries has scientific technology progressed to the point where we are able to separate the specific biochemical and purely physical properties of medicinal agents from any religious explanation. Biblically, the only things on record as being taken by mouth are food and drink. (Please note: The *King James Version* uses the word "herbs" to refer to plant foods, particularly vegetables. When we refer to herbs here, we are speaking of plants that appear to have specific medicinal purposes and are not meant to replace food.)

The very fact that certain plants have medicinal and/or druglike effects makes one wonder if God did not provide them for these very purposes. For example, in 1780, William Withering sent an elderly woman with congestive heart failure home to die. When he saw her later with her health much improved, he inquired as to the reason. She informed him that she'd begun using an herb called foxglove. Curious, Withering began to experiment, eventually isolating the substance we still use today for heart disease—digitalis (which stimulates stronger contraction and improved nerve transmission in the heart).[3] Opium also has no nutritional value, but specific receptors in the brain bind to these morphinelike substances for pain relief. Finally, banning all oral agents would clearly result in the needless deaths of countless numbers of people who depend upon them for their very lives. How could a caring physician deny lifesaving penicillin to a child with meningitis or withhold insulin from a juvenile onset diabetic?

Obviously these issues are quite complex and deserve a much more indepth discussion than we are able to provide within the context of this book. With regard to how herbs are taken, they are typically available in tinctures or capsules. A standard herbal infusion involves taking a pint of boiling water, pouring it over one ounce of ground herbs or roots and allowing it to steep for 5 to 15 minutes. A typical recommendation is to drink from one to three cups daily, as needed.

EVALUATING THROUGH THE GRID OF SCIENCE

Herbs and Drugs Are Different

Just like digitalis and morphine, many prescription drugs are direct or modified isolates from plants. Here are some of the advantages and disadvantages of using herbs rather than pharmaceutical drugs:

1. Herbs tend to have a higher *safety profile* than drugs. While herbs can cause toxicity, it is relatively uncommon.[4] Nevertheless, it does occur, so those who use herbs should do so with the same caution that needs to be exercised when taking pharmaceutical drugs.[5] In general, herbs should be used for specific conditions, limited periods of time and with the advice and counsel of someone who is knowledgeable in their use.

2. Active ingredients found in herbs occur in their *natural state*. This is a main reason why herbs tend to be less toxic and have fewer side effects. By contrast, pharmaceutical companies purposefully alter substances from their naturally occurring states in order to be able to patent the product as their own.

3. Herbs may contain important and yet still unknown *cofactors* that synthesized drugs do not. For example, once vitamin C was identified as an important natural antioxidant, it was synthesized in the laboratory and marketed as a supplement. Since then, numerous cofactors such as bioflavonoids have been discovered that greatly enhance the performance of vitamin C. But prior to their discovery, these important cofactors could only be obtained from their natural sources. Pharmaceutical agents will always have this limitation where nature does not.

4. Herbs tend to be *less expensive,* particularly when one considers the cost of doctor visits to obtain prescriptions. However, with rising costs in the alternative-health-products industry, this is not always the case. Furthermore, this advantage is insignificant if one is unknowingly treating a condition that truly needs a doctor's care. Indeed, this is one of the risks of self-medicating. Often independent individuals do not really know what they are treating and run the risk of denying themselves needed medical care or doing something that may worsen their condition.

5. One significant reason for the lower cost of herbs is that there is much *less research* associated with them. First, they are naturally occurring substances and are not discovered and developed in a research laboratory. Second, far fewer clinical studies tend to be done on herbs, leaving us relatively in the dark as to just how effective they really are.

6. Several years ago, I (Michael) put my wife on an herbal form of wild yam root with the (false) understanding that this product would naturally raise her levels of progesterone. Sometime later, we discovered through the services of a specialty laboratory that the product she was taking was "spiked" with a synthetic form of progesterone. This reveals another potential downside to herbs. Some have a reputation for *poor quality control* and *product integrity*. Government agencies such as the FDA maintain strict standards that pharmaceutical companies must follow in the preparation of their products. But at present, the same standards are not applied to the herbal and supplement industry.[6] Therefore, it is difficult to know from one herbal preparation to the next just how much active ingredient one is getting. This is generally not the case with pharmaceutical drugs, which have earned a reputation for reliability and consistency, if for no other reason than that the FDA watches them like a hawk.

> Herbs are naturally occurring substances and are not discovered and developed in a research laboratory.

Herbs Are Not Homeopathic Remedies

It is common today for people to incorrectly refer to herbs as homeopathic remedies and vice versa. Chapter 13, on homeopathy, states clearly that there is a vast difference between the two.[7] Homeopathic remedies may be derived from herbs or a variety of organic or inorganic sources, including minerals, drugs, venoms, animal secretions, etc. Furthermore, in order to be classified as homeopathic remedies, these substances must be prepared according to standard homeopathic methods. Their potencies are most often in infinitesimal doses.

Supplements Are on the Rise

It is not uncommon for me (Michael) to receive personal letters from individuals who are convinced of the effectiveness of a particular product and desire my endorsement. The letter usually includes an offer to "sign on" with them and recommend their product line so that together we might reap big dividends while helping others in the process. Even though I may appreciate the value of various products, I have purposed to avoid becoming financially involved in them in order to avoid the possibility of undermining our ministry by having our motives questioned.

Usually such correspondence is accompanied by impressive product literature, well laid out and filled with testimonials and claims that this particular company manufactures the best available—and perhaps only reliable—supplements on Earth. Last year, I got a letter that really took the cake. For our purposes, I have changed the name of the product to TooGoodToBeTrue.

> Fortunately, Mother Nature has provided us with a natural solution to stress known as adaptogens. Considered the number one stress reliever in the world, TooGoodToBeTrue was adaptogenically developed and tested for 45 years by Dr. (name withheld) and a team of Russian scientists in the former Soviet Union at an estimated cost of $1,000,000,000. Since then 1,200 scientists in more than 3,000 clinical studies have substantiated the effectiveness of TooGoodToBeTrue on stress in tens of thousands of Russian citizens.

Obviously, something is a little amiss. First, I have been to Russia and seen their health care. I can assure you that if there were 1 billion dollars available, it would not be spent on researching a nutritional supplement. Even the cost of developing a state-of-the-art drug by a top-notch pharmaceutical company in the U.S. is dwarfed by that figure. Second, where have you ever heard of even the best of drugs being researched by over 1,200 scientists in 3,000 clinical studies and in "tens of thousands" of subjects? The vast majority of studies that we have cited in this book involved less than 100 people. It just doesn't happen—it's too good to be true.

Claims such as these help point out that supplements have some of the same strengths and weaknesses as we see with herbs. But before we get into them, let's address what supplements are. A little history of how they first came to be will help.

Up until the eighteenth century, scurvy was a recurring problem among sailors who spent long periods away at sea. In 1757, James Lind discovered that this dreaded disease could be prevented by a regular intake of fresh fruit.[8] Likewise, Kanehiro Takaki (1849-1915), surgeon general of the Japanese Navy, realized that adding meat and vegetables to the diet of naval crews greatly reduced the number of beriberi cases.[9] A short time later, a Dutch medical officer named Christiaan Eijkman demonstrated that people who ate whole-grain rice were protected from beriberi, while those who ate polished rice were not. Casimir Funk (1884-1967) tried to isolate the anti-beriberi factor, but did not succeed. Nevertheless, the name he gave it, *vitamine*, stuck (he thought the substance, later identified as *thiamine*, was an amine, and that it was vital to life, thus the name vitamine). In

Supplements should be used to augment a good diet, not to replace one.

the 1900s, ascorbate (vitamin C) was identified as the ingredient within fruit responsible for its protective effect against scurvy. Once this discovery was made, techniques were developed to extract vitamin C from its natural sources and to concentrate it into capsules and tablets, which could be conveniently taken in much larger doses than ordinary food intake allowed.

As mentioned earlier, supplements carry with them some of the same strengths and weaknesses we noted with herbs. Despite the obvious fact that they are quite safe, toxicity can occur, particularly with especially large doses.[10] In addition, supplements lack unknown and, yet, probably important cofactors present in the natural food source.[11] They also tend to have a reputation for poor quality control. Many companies manufacture their products without clinically testing them to ensure that they are adequately digested, absorbed and utilized. For example, only 20 percent of magnesium oxide is absorbed from the intestines as compared to over 90 percent of magnesium when it is given in the malate form.

One final thing to bear in mind—supplements should be used to augment a good diet, not to replace one. They are supplements—not substitutes. Research has consistently affirmed that those who enjoy the best health get their nutrients principally from a wholesome, balanced diet, not from a box or jar. No supplement can make up for a bad diet. So enjoy the good food God gave you and supplement according to your specific needs.

Herbs and Supplements Possess Many Benefits

Numerous other books comprehensively address the value of specific vitamins, minerals and herbs. Therefore, what follows is a brief summarized list of those herbs and supplements that have some degree of research supporting their use in specific clinical indications.[12]

Athlete's foot: tea tree oil

Benign prostatic hypertrophy (BPH): saw palmetto and zinc

Burns: aloe, topical St. John's wort and witch hazel

Cancer prevention: nutrition, selenium, vitamin C and vitamin E

Cholesterol: nutrition, red yeast rice, chromium, evening primrose oil and garlic

Claudication: gingko biloba

Colds: echinacea, zinc and vitamin C

Colic: chamomile

Colitis: evening primrose oil

Constipation: aloe, diet and nutrition and senna

Depression: light therapy, St. John's wort and evening primrose oil

Diabetes: diet and nutrition, chromium, ginseng, bilberry, burdock and evening primrose oil

Diarrhea: bilberry

Eczema: evening primrose oil

Fibromyalgia: willow bark and honeybee venom

Flu: echinacea and elderberry

Fungal nail infections: topical tea tree oil

Headache: gingko biloba and willow bark

Heart disease: nutrition, hawthorn, evening primrose oil, ginseng, grape seed extract and vitamin E

Heart failure: coenzyme Q10, ginseng

Hemorrhoids: senna, witch hazel

Hepatitis: milk thistle, licorice

High blood pressure: diet and nutrition, coenzyme Q10 and garlic

Hot flashes: black cohosh

Insect bites: aloe and marigold

Insomnia: valerian, chamomile and ginseng

Macular degeneration: bilberry

Memory loss: gingko biloba and ginseng

Menstrual problems and menopause: black cohosh

Migraine: feverfew and willow bark

Neuropathy: topical capsaicin and evening primrose oil

Peripheral artery disease: gingko biloba

Psoriasis: light therapy and capsaicin

Respiratory problems: licorice

Rheumatoid arthritis: evening primrose oil, willow bark, ginger, glucosamine, honeybee venom and zinc

Sore throat: bilberry and slippery elm

Tinnitus: gingko biloba

Urinary tract infections: cranberry

EVALUATING THROUGH THE GRID OF SPIRITUAL DISCERNMENT

In general, the use of vitamins, minerals, herbs and prescription medications do not, in and of themselves, impinge upon the spiritual realm except when their effects become toxic, when they significantly alter the mind or when they are used as part of a religious and/or psychic experience.

CONCLUSION

Whether an herb, drug or food supplement, all need to be considered medicinal agents of one degree or another and, therefore, used with some degree of caution. While there is little biblical basis for putting anything other than food and drink in your mouth, we have attempted to leave room for the value and appropriateness of these potential remedies. Each has its own purpose, but cannot and should not displace the value of a prudent, balanced diet and other lifestyle measures. These, in most cases, are the only truly legitimate long-term solutions.

CHAPTER NINETEEN

CHELATION, MAGNETS AND TOUCH THERAPIES

CHELATION

Evaluating Through the Grids of History, Faith and Wholism

Chelation therapy has been around since the 1940s. Apparently, its first clinical use was by the United States Navy to treat lead poisoning. During the 1950s, some patients being treated with chelation for lead poisoning reported that their angina (chest pain from heart disease) improved. This led Dr. Norman Clarke, Sr., of Detroit, Michigan, to propose that chelation therapy be used to treat heart disease. Ever since, practitioners have used it for not only clogged arteries, but for almost every conceivable chronic disease.[1]

Chelation comes from the Greek word *chele*, meaning "claw." In medicine, the term is used to refer to the way in which chelators bind heavy metals, grasping them at multiple points like a giant claw and escorting them to the kidney where they are excreted in the urine. Heavy metals (such as lead, silver, mercury, aluminum, etc.) are not believed to be involved in normal body function. They can become toxic to humans in at least two ways.

1. **Oxidative stress.** Heavy metals have strong positive charges that tend to pull electrons from other compounds, thus oxidizing them. Substances with unpaired electrons are referred to as free radicals.

These are known to cause significant damage to body tissues. They also oxidize LDL cholesterol into its most harmful form.

2. **Binding enzymes.** Minerals and enzymes work together to perform many critical functions in the body. For example, selenium is a cofactor for the enzyme that is responsible for the conversion of the T4 thyroid hormone into its more active T3 form. Zinc is critical for the proper function of superoxide dismutase (SOD), a frontline defense that neutralizes free radicals. Heavy metals, such as lead, mercury, arsenic and others can potentially interfere with the binding of these enzymes to their proper cofactors and, therefore, interfere with their functioning.[2]

In order to remove heavy metals from the body, a variety of chelating agents are used, both orally and intravenously. The most common chelating agent used is ethylenediaminetetraacetic acid (EDTA). A typical treatment course involves anywhere from 6 to 40 treatments over several weeks to months. Since EDTA is ineffective against mercury (in fact, it may even cause harm to nerve tissue if it binds with mercury),[3] other agents, such as d-penicillamine and 2,3-dimercapto-1-propanesulfonate (DMPS) are used to eliminate this heavy metal.[4] Here are some examples of how and why chelation is used in alternative therapy.

1. **Multiple sclerosis** involves injury and/or destruction of the myelin sheath that envelops nerves. Some believe that this damage is due to the oxidizing effects of heavy metals. Chelation is given to remove heavy metals from the body and to reduce the "oxidative burden."

2. **Coronary artery disease (CAD)** is caused by a buildup of plaque, which is a firm, rubbery substance that consists of calcium and cholesterol compounds. Proponents used to claim that chelation pulled calcium out of plaque, making it softer and more amenable to breakdown by the body. However, this theory has largely been supplanted by newer explanations, such as the ability of EDTA to reduce oxidative burden and, thereby, protect LDL cholesterol from being oxidized—a key step in the development of plaque.[5]

3. **Various other diseases,** including Alzheimer's disease, amyotrophic lateral sclerosis (ALS, Lou Gehrig's disease), infertility, Parkinson's disease, etc.

4. **Mercury toxicity** in patients who have received dental amalgam fillings (the standard silver color), often use chelation as a preventative treatment.[6]

Evaluating Through the Grid of Science

The value of chelation therapy in treating heavy-metal toxicity has been unquestionably proven. In this regard, particularly with respect to lead toxicity, chelation is not considered an alternative treatment. It is mainstream allopathic medicine.[7] However, beyond that, the controversy begins, and trying to find consensus appears near to impossible.

In Brazil, a clinic reviewed nearly 3,000 charts, claiming that chelation improved symptoms in the vast majority of their patients suffering from a variety of diseases.[8] However, the fact remains that there is almost no reliable evidence (i.e., well-designed research studies) to support the use of chelation therapy in the treatment of anything other than heavy-metal toxicity. For example, with regard to chelation as a treatment for blocked arteries in the legs, a 1997 comprehensive search of medical literature found only four randomized, placebo-controlled, double-blind trials. While one poor-quality study indicated that chelation might help, the other three (which were all assessed as of outstanding quality) concluded that EDTA chelation was no better than placebo.[9] (See table B-6 for further discussion on this study.)

Many in alternative health care attribute allopathic medicine's opposition to chelation to a closed-minded, money-hungry, medical profession that is purposefully withholding this lifesaving treatment from patients. Common sense should tell you that that is highly unlikely. First of all, chelation is very compatible with an allopathic paradigm. There is no good reason to reject it from a philosophical standpoint. Second, chelation is a medical procedure. It requires a doctor to prescribe it, and since there are so many people with diseases that should supposedly benefit from it, doctors could earn a lot of money doing it. Third, with as many people as there are who do have chelation each year, it should be obvious that if it were a miracle cure, it would be clearly known as such by now. We truly wish it were what its proponents claim it to be. But from all we can tell, it is not.

However, you have probably met or heard of people with heart problems who claim to have personally benefited from chelation therapy. Perhaps one reason for the confusion is that chelation is often mixed with other forms of treatment. For example, some alternative practitioners give vitamins and minerals intravenously in conjunction with a chelation protocol. One study showed that when EDTA chelation was given with vitamin B, it improved the ability of blood vessels to "relax" and "open up," but not when EDTA was given alone.[10] Therefore, in some cases at least, if there truly is a benefit beyond the placebo effect, it may be due to nutritional therapy, not the chelating agent.

Mercury and dental amalgam. Mercury toxicity (or the concern of it) is probably the second most common reason for why patients seek chelation. As with the heart disease controversy, there is considerable debate within the dental profession as to whether or not mercury is a significant source of toxicity in human beings. Mercury is the largest ingredient in dental amalgam, accounting for approximately 50 percent of its contents.[11] The American Dental Association (ADA) has taken a firm stand for decades on this issue, maintaining that there is insufficient evidence to implicate mercury amalgam as a significant contributor to human toxicity and disease.[12] Consistent with its position, the ADA has declared it unethical for its members to arbitrarily recommend removal of amalgam fillings merely on the basis of toxicity concerns.[13]

However, there are highly credible voices that strongly disagree with the ADA; most significantly, the International Academy of Oral Medicine and Toxicology (IAOMT). The IAOMT has gathered a significant body of research in coming to its conclusion that dental amalgam, and mercury in particular, are potentially serious health threats. Their presentations before national governments have been persuasive enough that standard amalgam fillings are now banned in Germany.[14] Dr. Hal Huggins frames the debate with four fundamental questions.[15]

1. **Does mercury leak from dental fillings?** The answer to this question is an unequivocal yes. The amount of mercury in the urine in the average individual correlates more closely with the number of fillings they have than with any other factor, including fish intake.[16]
2. **Does mercury form a toxic compound?** Again, an unequivocal yes. Mercury is vaporized from dental amalgam during chewing and then inhaled where it deposits in tissue.[17]
3. **Does it form enough of this compound to produce illness?** Here is where there is some question. More than one study indicates that

mercury amalgam can cause lichenoid deposits (hard white streaks) on the inside of the mouth, which disappear once the fillings are removed. In addition, a female dentist experienced symptoms of Parkinson's disease that immediately and permanently cleared after she received chelation treatment. On the flip side, Canadian dentists who are exposed to mercury every day at work do not have a shorter life expectancy than nondentists. Other studies have found that the amount of mercury in a person does correlate with the number of fillings they have, but does not correlate with the number of symptoms they have. Furthermore, several studies found that the only health problems that correlated with the number of dental fillings, or mercury, in the body were psychological, leading the authors to conclude that mercury toxicity from amalgam was due to patients' fear and imagination.[18]

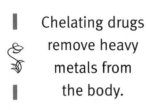 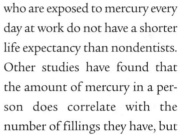

Chelating drugs remove heavy metals from the body.

4. **Can illness be reduced or eliminated by amalgam removal (or chelation)?** In most people, probably not. Mercury levels dramatically fall after removal of amalgam. However, while some studies show a correlation between mercury and disease, such as Alzheimer's, Parkinson's and multiple sclerosis, we were unable to find clinical trials that actually showed that a particular disease would improve or be reversed after amalgam removal and/or chelation.[19]

Evaluating Through the Grid of Spiritual Discernment

There does not seem to be any spirit-realm involvement inherent to chelation therapy. It appears to be a purely physical-realm issue.

Conclusion

Chelating drugs remove heavy metals from the body. Chelation works, there is no question about that. The questions are whether or not heavy metals are causing these diseases and whether or not chelating the metals will result in improvement or cure. Because there are so few actual clinical trials that have examined this, we just can't say at this point. If you are considering chelation, we recommend several things. First, get a thorough evaluation prior to initiating therapy, so you and your doctor know what your current condition is. Second, get tested for heavy metals (blood and/or urine) prior to and periodically while undergoing chelation. Third, stay under the care of your conventional doctor, who can monitor your condition. Fourth, be as objective as you can as to whether or not the treatment is really helping. Fifth, make necessary lifestyle changes to more effectively address your problem from a long-term perspective. You should not have to keep going back for treatments indefinitely.

MAGNETS

Michael had a friend who told me that he might need some help rearranging his bedroom furniture. He explained that one of his health-care providers had recommended that he optimize his health by turning his bed so that while he slept he would be aligned with the magnetic north and south poles. Would this have a significant effect on him?

Evaluating Through the Grid of History

Magnetic therapy traces its roots to Frank Anton Mesmer, an eighteenth-century Austrian physician who was discussed in chapter 7. Mesmer believed that life and health come from an invisible energy called *anima* and that aberrations in this energy flow resulted in disease. These aberrations could, according to Mesmer, be corrected with the use of magnetic therapy. While he initially used magnets to treat patients, eventually he came to believe that doctors could serve as mediums, transmitting their own magnetic energy ("animal magnetism") to their patients. During treatment sessions, his patients went into a trance; in other words, they became mesmerized. Thus, hypnosis also attributes its start in Western medicine to Mesmer.[20]

Magnetic therapy has since experienced brief periods of resurgence in popularity, only to fall away into obscurity for another season. Regardless of whether those who utilized magnetic therapy were applying magnets to their patients or mesmerizing them, this healing profession was still considered outside the mainstream medical practice. Recently, the use of magnets has once again become popular in and outside of the U.S. This resurgence in popularity is a result of aggressive marketing strategies by magnet manufacturers coupled with a greater interest in alternative healing approaches.

Evaluating Through the Grid of Faith

As noted above, Mesmer believed that magnets (including the magnetic capacity of the healer) could be used to correct aberrations in the flow of the health-giving life force. Life-force concepts, as explained in other parts of this book, originated in Eastern religious systems. Therefore, it should be no surprise that the major manufacturer for magnet products is based in the Orient. Obviously, Mesmer's worldview included this life-force concept, as is indicated by both his use of the term *anima* and his willingness to serve as a medium in which the doctor's appointment bears a closer resemblance to a séance.

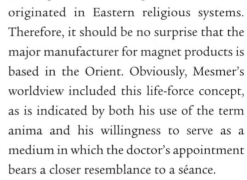

> Manufacturers have designed magnetic products for every conceivable need, including mattresses, seat pads, necklaces, shoe inserts and even horse blankets.

On the other hand, using magnets in medicine does not necessarily imply that one has embraced Eastern or New Age premises. Magnets are physical objects with physical properties. They are used in medicine every day in a variety of applications without our ever thinking of a moral or spiritual implication, such as in magnetic resonance imaging (MRI).

Evaluating Through the Wholistic Grid

There are three general approaches to magnetic therapy in medicine. Due to its popularity within the Church, we will focus the majority of our attention on the third category.

1. **Psychic.** As noted above, Mesmer eventually gravitated toward the use of psychic healing, believing that the doctor functions as a medium for magnetic healing to his or her patients.

2. **Pulsating magnetic therapy.** Since Michael Faraday's experiments, which demonstrated passing an electrical current through a coil to produce a magnetic field, researchers have considered the possible beneficial effects this might have on the human frame. Recently, pulsating electromagnetic therapy has been used to stimulate repair of bone fractures, particularly those that have failed to heal adequately.[21]

3. **Permanent magnets.** This involves the direct application of Magnets to the body. For example, for someone with chronic lower-back pain, a pair of magnets might be applied to the skin on either side of the area of pain, much like electrodes of a transcutaneous electrical nerve stimulator (TENS) unit. Manufacturers have designed magnetic products for every conceivable need, including mattresses, seat pads, necklaces, shoe inserts and even horse blankets.

Evaluating Through the Grid of Science

Of the three types of magnetic therapy, only the second appears to show much legitimate promise. According to Doctors O'Mathúna and Larimore, the pulsating magnetic therapy is legitimate because a magnetic field must pulsate in order for voltage to be produced. They claim, "There is no known way for a permanent magnet to induce electrical current."[22] In other words, fixed magnets should not work. Indeed, the evidence seems to confirm this. A review of the website for perhaps the largest medical magnet manufacturer in the world produced no scientific citations to support its use. (For a comprehensive search of the National Library of Medicine for clinical trials utilizing permanent magnets, please refer to table B-7.) In summary, relatively little scientific evidence apparently exists to support magnetic therapy.

Evaluating Through the Grid of Spiritual Discernment

When permanent magnets or pulsating magnetic fields are used strictly for their biophysical properties, they can be evaluated strictly on the basis of their scientific validity. However, when the basis for the use of magnetic therapy implies manipulation of some form of life force, its use should be seriously questioned. Moreover, Mesmer's concept of the doctor as medium clearly involves contact with the occult and should be completely avoided.

While objective studies on the use of magnets in their popular form indicate that they probably don't work, they are probably not harmful when worn for brief periods of time, especially away from the head. However, we do wonder about the long-term effects of constant exposure to magnetic fields (though the fields are probably weak to nonexistent), especially when magnets are placed on the head or when exposed to magnets while lying on an object such as a mattress. However, there are no long-term studies yet.

TOUCH THERAPIES

Evaluating Through the Grid of History

Touching people to help them get well has probably been around since man first became sick. It is central to several healing techniques and systems such as osteopathy, chiropractic and multiple forms of massage therapy.

According to historians, a variation of the therapeutic laying on of hands has been around for almost as long. These are the energy-based approaches to touching, or should we say, nontouching. Among these include: healing touch, therapeutic touch, polarity, reiki, jin shin jyutsu, external qigong, Touch For Health, reflexology, acupressure and shiatsu massage. Several of these are addressed elsewhere in this book. This chapter will focus on the two most popular approaches in America, both of which came into the health-care system via the nursing profession.

Delores Krieger, a professor of nursing at New York University, introduced the first approach, known as therapeutic touch (TT), in a 1975 journal article. Krieger became interested in using touch as a means of healing through studying the writings of a Hungarian healer named Oskar Estebany. Later, she was tutored under Dora Kunz, who at that time served as president of the Theosophical Society in America, and who was said by Krieger to have been "born with a unique ability to perceive subtle energies around living beings."[23] Eventually, Krieger offered an elective course on therapeutic touch to nursing students and began teaching workshops nationwide.

Janet Mentgen, a Colorado nurse, developed the second approach. A practitioner of various energy-based touch therapies for years, Mentgen was eventually introduced to TT. Upon doing so, she combined TT with other approaches and referred to her own as healing touch (HT). In 1990, her own course was offered for certification by the American Holistic Nurses' Association (AHNA) as the healing touch for health care professionals. The AHNA also offers training in hypnosis for those who want to go beyond HT.[24]

Evaluating Through the Grid of Faith

Practically all energy-based touch therapies trace their philosophical roots and practices back to ancient India. Of therapeutic touch, one textbook writer says, "this is a type of pranic healing, a modern interpretation of several ancient healing practices, traditionally known as the 'laying on of hands.'"[25] Dora Kunz claimed that, "Healing energy is a beneficent power available to all living beings . . . (since) this healing power or energy is available to everyone, it is essentially the same, no matter how it may be described."[26]

In other words, practitioners of this approach speak in terms of energy; although, they use words such as "spirit" and "consciousness" interchangeably. Obviously, the underlying worldview has the same basis as that found in Eastern religions and medical practices.

Evaluating Through the Wholistic Grid

When Western medical practitioners seek to include other dimensions of reality into their therapeutic practices, they seem to gravitate toward Eastern religions. That has not been true for the West. Even though Christianity has been the major religious choice in America and Europe, Christians haven't sought to integrate their worldview into their Christian medical practices, other than their concern for ethics and the pastoral care of the sick.

Although each of these touch-energy approaches possess unique qualities, their similarities are far greater than their differences. A typical TT session involves the following steps:

1. **Centering.** The practitioner utilizes a personal form of meditation in an attempt to come to a place of mental rest along with an "intention to heal."

2. **Scanning.** The hands are usually placed several inches above the patient as the practitioner tunes in to their client's energy field to detect any abnormalities. According to this theory, a healthy individual will have a smooth uniform energy pattern that flows like an unhindered river. On the other hand, those who are sick will have disruptions in their energy pattern with temperature fluctuations or senses of stagnation, heaviness, holes, leaks, etc.

3. **Unruffling.** Once disturbances are identified, the practitioner attempts to "unruffle" the energy disturbance and smooth it out, either by using sweeps of the hands or by mentally directing energy to where it is needed. Sessions usually last from 5 to 30 minutes.[27]

Reiki. Reiki is another version of a hand-mediated energy healing technique. It traces its roots to a nineteenth-century Japanese Zen Buddhist monk, Mikao

Usui. On a search to learn how to recreate the healing miracles of Jesus Christ, Usui experienced a trance state while on a three-week fast on Mount Koriyama. There he claimed to have discovered the secret to healing and called it reiki.[28]

Reiki comes from two Japanese words. The first, *rei*, meaning universal, refers to the highest form of wisdom, supernatural knowledge or consciousness. It is the God-consciousness that knows each person's need. This ultimate source of life energy is available to all along with its unconditional love and healing power. The second word is *ki*, the Japanese term for qi, which is the life force. According to this theory, rei, the God-consciousness, directs the life force ki, in the practice of reiki. The practitioner functions as a medium or conduit for ki energy to the patient.[29] Since the God-consciousness knows the patient's needs, the practitioner is not to attempt to influence the treatment.

Similar to a therapeutic touch session, the practitioner places his or her hands a few inches above the patient and waits for energy flow to begin. After an average of five minutes, the hands are moved sequentially through each of the other dozen positions, each being held for an average of five minutes. Thus, a total treatment session usually lasts about one hour.

Reiki practitioners go through extensive training. At each level, students supposedly receive a bolus of life energy from their reiki master. To become a first-degree reiki practitioner, the student must be able to detect and move life energy. To achieve second-degree, one must be able to send life energy over longer distances. The third and final level is that of a reiki master, an elite group whose membership is by invitation only.

Evaluating Through the Grid of Science

Massage therapies have been studied quite extensively and have been shown to have beneficial effects in a number of conditions. Gentle stroking has improved the health and shortened hospital stays of premature newborns, which points to the need of human beings to be touched. Massage has also been shown to be helpful in relieving stress and anxiety, and in helping patients to relax. Because of its ability to help stimulate circulation, it has also been shown to promote healing and relieve soreness and pain.[30]

Touch is also central to the osteopathic and chiropractic systems. However, these systems apply to more developed concepts with the goal of correcting structural malpositions, relieving stress on strained ligaments and improving circulation and nerve transmission.

Energy-based approaches such as HT and TT do not enjoy the same degree of scientific credibility. About half of the research studies appear to show some potential benefit (usually in relation to the same kinds of things noted for massage therapy), while the other half indicate that they are of little or no value.

The most famous clinical study was the idea of a nine-year-old fourth-grade student named Emily Rosa. The daughter of a nurse who objected to therapeutic touch, Emily wondered if TT practitioners could actually sense the human energy field. Therefore, as a science class project, she enlisted the services of 15 TT practitioners who agreed to participate. Each practitioner was sequentially seated at a table behind a cardboard screen that included cutouts through which the therapist would insert his or her arms. Emily sat on the other side of the screen where she flipped a coin to decide which of the practitioner's hands would be chosen. Once determined, Emily held her hand a few inches above the selected hand of the practitioner who was given as much time as desired to determine which of the practitioner's own hands was the one under Emily's hand. Each practitioner was given multiple tries.

Of 150 attempts, the TT practitioners were only correct in 71, which amounted to 47 percent. Since with each attempt the therapist had a 50-50 chance of being right, TT practitioners fared no better than random guessing. The following year, the entire experiment was replicated with 13 practitioners as part of a Public Broadcasting System feature. This time, therapeutic touch did even worse, with a success rate of only 41 percent. With the assistance of Stephen Barrett, M.D., Emily's experiment was submitted to and published on April Fools' Day 1998.[31] (See table B-8 for a summarized list of touch therapy clinical trials. We were able to find no clinical trials testing the effectiveness of reiki. Even if we had, we would have to question which spirit was at work.)

Evaluating Through the Grid of Spiritual Discernment

Many proponents of energy-based touch therapies openly acknowledge that these practices involve either manipulation of energy "life force" or overt

> Many proponents of energy-based touch therapies openly acknowledge that these practices involve either manipulation of energy "life force" or overt spiritual forces.

spiritual forces. In some, the practice is claimed to involve the healer serving as a medium or conduit on behalf of the patient. It seems obvious that there may be involvement in the spiritual realm, and it is unlikely to be the Holy Spirit.

CONCLUSION

Healing touch, therapeutic touch and other related energy-based approaches are now in common use. They claim to have trained over 100,000 practitioners, particularly through their wholesale acceptance into the nursing profession. Proponents enthusiastically affirm their use on medical wards, labor and delivery units and Lamaze classes across the country. Perhaps of greatest concern is their practice in places where patients or guardians may not have the choice to decline, such as in newborn nurseries, recovery rooms, pediatric wards and psychiatric units. From a biblical perspective, we have strong cautions regarding these approaches.

We also believe this is a spiritual counterfeit. As mentioned earlier in the book, touch is an important part of Christianity. We encourage parents to gently lay hands on their children and pray for their health and protection. We regularly hold hands when we pray. We believe in the personal presence of God within us. We extend our hands toward others when we pray. We are not trying to project some human or impersonal energy, we are extending our hearts in identification to one another. The bond is the omnipresent Holy Spirit who indwells us. He is the One who draws us together, who binds up the brokenhearted and sets the captives free.

CHAPTER TWENTY

MIND-BODY MEDICINE

A sound heart is the life of the flesh.

PROVERBS 14:30, *KJV*

If you were to ask her, Candice would say that the most powerful physical heal-ing agent available is not a drug; it is a sound (healthy) spiritual heart and mind. As a 50-year-old pastor's wife, Candice was given the devastating diagnosis of metastatic breast cancer. By the time it was discovered, the disease had already spread throughout her body, and she was given only a few months to live. In response to her diagnosis, she and her husband sought the counsel of a Georgia pastor whose ministry orientation is in identifying spiritual factors in the cause of disease. During their conversation, Candice became aware of the possibility that bitterness toward another woman had weakened her immune system and made her more vulnerable to cancer. Shortly thereafter, she sought forgiveness and was reconciled in her relationship with the woman from whom she had been estranged. That was four years ago. As of this writing, her cancer has spontaneously regressed despite the fact that she has never changed her diet, has never had surgery and has not taken any medications. She still has no symp-toms and feels great.

Jane could also testify to the power of a sound heart and mind. After deliv-ering her second child, she developed a psychosis and lost touch with reality. During the course of her illness, friends counseled and supported her in prayer. During one particular visit, a friend shared with her the devastating effects of bitterness in one's life. As she shared, Jane recalled being abused when she was a young girl, a memory that she had repressed for many years. As she recalled the event, she realized she had never forgiven her offender for what he had done. When she confessed her bitterness and forgave him, her psychosis began to clear. As two other unresolved conflicts were identified, her thinking was eventually completely restored.

Scripture bears witness to the relationship that righteousness and a sound mind have with our physical health. David affirmed that a guilty conscience caused his body to waste away (see Ps. 32:1-5). Nabal, one of David's enemies, experienced the devastating effects of a violated conscience in much more dramatic fashion. When his wife told him that she had interceded for his life before David (who was on his way to kill him in revenge for Nabal's mistreatment), Nabal's heart "became as a stone" and he died 10 days later (see 1 Sam. 25:37-38).

> The brain can only function according to how the mind has been programmed.

How is it that our minds can have such dramatic effects on our bodies? The answer in most cases is found in what medicine refers to as stress. Stress accounts for as much as 75 percent of all physician visits.[1] Recall from chapter 5 that the mind is what determines the signal that is sent to the adrenal glands, which in turn releases adrenaline and cortisol into our bloodstreams. Stress can have powerful negative influences on virtually every organ system in the body.[2] These physical effects were discussed in detail in *The Word on Health*.[3] Suffice it here to cite psychologist Archibald Hart, who said, "Stress begins in the mind but ends in the body . . . there is no such thing as stress only being in the mind."[4] Perhaps that is why there is such an emphasis in medicine on relaxation. The biblical ideal is for every child of God to have peace of mind and rest for their soul.

APPROACHING MIND-BODY MEDICINE

Mind-body medicine usually takes on three different forms. The first is passive in nature and usually emphasizes relaxation. Calming one's thoughts and emotions not only refreshes the soul, but it also has physical benefits, because it reduces the release of adrenaline and other components of the fight-or-flight system that becomes activated during stress.[5]

The most common passive mind-body approach today is meditation, which was discussed in chapter 9. Another common modality is visualization, in which the individual seeks a comfortable position and pictures a peaceful scene or environment in order to become relaxed. Biofeedback also adds to visualization, which is the use of instruments to give feedback on the activity of various body processes, such as heart and breathing rates, blood pressure, skin temperature (an indirect measurement of blood flow), muscle tension and so on. Again, all of these are regulated by the autonomic nervous system, which plays a preeminent role in how the body handles stress.[6] Additionally, the autonomic nervous system is regulated by the central nervous system (brain and spinal cord), and that is affected by what we believe. Recall that the brain can only function according to how the mind has been programmed.

Most Western scientists used to believe that the parameters controlled by the autonomic nervous system were beyond the realm of conscious control. But research has indicated that some individuals can use biofeedback and other methods in a more active mode—to focus thoughts in such a way as to specifically influence certain body processes (e.g., slow the heart rate down, lower blood pressure, etc.). In a general sense, we have all used our minds to control body functions, the most obvious of which is the somatic nervous system (i.e., muscular movements). First, we can't do anything without first thinking it. Second, when we find ourselves stressed out or anxious, we tell ourselves to calm down, get a grip, put it in perspective, and so on. Managing our thoughts has enabled us to slow down, relax and "chill out" (as our children have counseled us more than once). This results in a reduction in autonomic nervous system activity.

Guided imagery is the second approach—another active process—which directs our minds in order to affect our autonomic nervous system. In this case, the imagination (i.e., thought) is used to assist or accomplish a specific health or medical purpose. For example, cancer patients may be encouraged to visualize chemotherapy drugs traveling to the cancer site and destroying malignant cells. Using the imagination in this way is believed by some to enhance the effects of medications or to strengthen the body's immune system as it attacks and destroys these cells.

The third approach in mind-body medicine involves yielding control (at least partially) of one's mind to that of another. This approach is utilized in hypnosis and various psychic practices. Hypnosis is defined as "an artificially induced passive state in which there is increased amenability and responsiveness to suggestions and commands, provided that these do not conflict seriously with the subject's own conscious or unconscious wishes."[7]

The first use of hypnosis in medicine is attributed to Frank Mesmer, who was discussed in chapter 7. Known initially as mesmerism, it was eventually given the name hypnosis by James Braid (1795-1860), an English physician who gave mesmerism an alias in order to disconnect the practice from its tainted reputation and founder.[8] In Western medicine, hypnosis is most commonly employed for the relief or prevention of pain. It is also used as an anesthesia. Psychology also utilizes it as an aid in recovering repressed memories and addressing personality types in dissociative disorders. Some therapists have used it to enhance performance and to overcome bad habits.

EVALUATING THROUGH THE GRID OF SCIENCE

Does research validate mind-body medicine in its various forms, such as biofeedback, visualization, guided imagery and hypnosis? The answer is yes and no. Biofeedback has been shown in numerous scientific studies to be fairly effective in helping people relax. Therefore, it is considered medically useful in relieving anxiety as well as reducing blood pressure and certain types of pain, particularly headaches.[9] However, it is not a cure in and of itself, but rather, a means of coping with symptoms such as those just described. The faith of the client is usually not being challenged in mind-body medical practices, only the use of the mind to affect the body.

Similarly, meditation and visualization have also been shown to be effective in helping people relax.[10] Nevertheless, there is little credible scientific data to suggest that active techniques such as guided imagery accomplish anything more than relaxation. No substantial evidence exists to support claims that it enhances the immune system or the performance of chemotherapy drugs.

Finally, while there are some studies that seem to indicate that hypnosis is effective as a substitute for pain medication or anesthesia, many others conclude exactly the opposite—that it doesn't work. In other words, there is no clear proof that hypnosis is a legitimate therapeutic approach. Furthermore, from a spiritual perspective, it is a highly questionable practice.

EVALUATING THROUGH THE
GRID OF SPIRITUAL DISCERNMENT

People normally visualize activities and have daydreams, often without even realizing it. While sitting at a desk, an executive daydreams about his family, a fishing trip or a desired position. A young bride-to-be pictures a home filled with love and the laughter of happy children. Children certainly have a reputation for possessing the most active imaginations. I (Michael) recall walking by the patio door years ago and noticing one of my sons outside playing alone. Totally engrossed in his own imaginary world, he watched himself in the reflection of the glass as he attacked the enemy, fought bravely, was mortally wounded and heroically died as he went through a series of magnificent contortions.

In sports, athletes attempt to improve their performance by visualizing perfect form prior to engaging in competition. For example, a golfer visualizes the perfect shot, first during a practice swing and then solely in his mind prior to addressing the ball. In this case, visualization is an attempt to recall and reinforce the complex stored memory pattern of a proper swing.

Few, if any, would find any spiritual danger in using their minds this way. Even attempts to use imagination to relax the body, such as in visualization or biofeedback, can function purely in the physical realm. However, some obviously take the idea of mind-body control well beyond these parameters. For example, visualization is commonly employed in Oriental medicine because of the underlying Eastern belief that man can create physical reality with his mind—what you think is what is real. This is similar to the belief held by Christian Science practitioners. They believe that all sickness is illusory—you're only sick because you believe you're sick (don't try telling that to someone who has just been hit by a car). Furthermore, some also use visualization to contact one's inner self, subconscious or spirit, which is also characteristic of some types of hypnosis.

Hypnosis has, since its inception, been consistently utilized by psychic and occult practitioners. Even so, despite this guilt by association and the fact that those under the power of hypnosis are significantly more open to suggestion, numerous Christians still advocate its use, insisting that it is a valuable mode of treatment. They assert that the cautions regarding hypnosis can be adequately addressed by simply providing an appropriate, protected environment. An appropriate environment typically means that the hypnotists are skilled practitioners who can be thoroughly trusted to not exploit the vulnerability of their patients. The protected environment, however, applies only in the physical realm.

But how does all of this line up with Scripture? Is it appropriate for Christians to practice hypnosis? To visualize? Does the Bible support altered states of consciousness? Are our thoughts to be controlled by the power of suggestion or by someone else? Is there a biblical basis for mind-body medicine?

EVALUATING THROUGH THE GRID OF FAITH

God often used "word pictures," a form of imagery, to communicate spiritual truth. Jesus likened the kingdom of God to leaven, a mustard seed, a costly pearl and a field of grain ready for harvest. He also spoke in parables—imaginary stories that He used to reveal (or conceal) spiritual principles. Jesus even used figurative speech when He referred to Himself as the Bread of Life, the light of the world, the rock, the Good Shepherd and the way, the truth and the life (see Ps. 19:14; Matt. 5:14; John 6:35; 10:11; 14:6). Christians are exhorted to consider (i.e., believe or think of) themselves as being dead to sin, crucified with Christ, buried with Him in His death, raised with Him in His resurrection and seated with Him in heavenly places (see Rom. 6:2-4; Gal. 2:20; Eph. 2:5-6). Mentally picturing a spiritual truth is a legitimate part of the Christian life.

The "eyes" of faith envision the reality of the spiritual world even though it is not visible to the natural eyes. Jesus said to the woman at the well, "God is a Spirit: and they that worship him must worship him in spirit and in truth" (John 4:24, *KJV*). Scripture is replete with examples of Jews and Christians interfacing in one form or another with the spiritual realm. God's people are encouraged to address Him through prayer, meditation, praise and worship. In addition, either directly or through angelic beings, God spoke on numerous occasions to individuals through dreams (such as with Abraham, Jacob, Joseph and Mary) and visions. In examples of the latter, individuals were even reported to go into trancelike states, such as when Peter "fell into a trance" while on the roof of the tanner's house in Joppa (Acts 10:10) or when Paul went into a trance while

> We are to maintain an active state of mind and direct our thoughts toward God.

praying in the Temple at Jerusalem (Acts 22:17). And in 2 Corinthians 12:1-4, Paul was caught up into the third heaven, whatever that is!

New Age practitioners who claim there is a biblical basis for guided imagery, visualization and other psychic powers often cite these kinds of references. In fact, many New Agers believe that Jesus was the first true psychic. However, a closer look at these Scriptures reveals some significant differences from the practices we find in New Age medicine.

1. In the Bible, a trance state was never sought. There is no evidence (other than with prayer, meditation and worship) to indicate that any of these biblical experiences were sought by the individual. Instead, they were obviously initiated by God.
2. There was no human intermediary. In no case was a human being involved who induced a trance state. When humans were involved, they were referred to as mediums and the practice was condemned.
3. Thought control was never surrendered to another being—human or spiritual.

An Active State of Mind

The Bible never instructs us to direct our thoughts inward, and we are never told to assume a passive state of the mind. We are to maintain an active state of mind and direct our thoughts toward God. We are instructed to invite God to examine us.

> Search me, O God, and know my heart; try me and know my anxious thoughts; and see if there be any hurtful way in me, and lead me in the everlasting way (Ps. 139:23-24).

God never bypasses our minds. When interacting with the spiritual world, Paul says, "I shall pray with the spirit and I shall pray with the mind also; I shall sing with the spirit and I shall sing with the mind also" (1 Cor. 14:15). This is one way to detect a counterfeit spirit. If the mind is being bypassed, it is a counterfeit. "Brethren, do not be children in your thinking; yet in evil be babes, but in your thinking be mature" (1 Cor. 14:20). We are transformed by the renewing of our minds (see Rom. 12:2), but we can also be destroyed by the depravity of our minds (see Rom. 1:28-32).

Passive thinking and mind control is actually being fostered in some of our churches. I (Neil) received the following letter from a lady who attended one of our conferences:

A committed Christian for many years, I was still having difficulty with some painful childhood memories caused by growing up in an abusive home. Several years ago, I attended an inner-healing seminar at my church to hopefully get some help.

Wanting all the Lord had for me, I fully participated in a guided-imagery session. The leader had the entire group close their eyes, quiet their minds with music and imagine that we climbed onto a magic carpet that took us to a beautiful meadow with a lake. She then led us into several imaginary events. I now know they were from the adversary.

Because of great turmoil in my life, and desperately needing help, I sought a pastor who led me through the Steps to Freedom in Christ.[11] It was an encounter with the awesome love of my heavenly Father like I've never experienced before.

At the beginning of the session, with the help of a loving, gentle pastor, the Lord revealed a spirit guide that had gained entrance during the inner-healing guided imagery. I had learned to look forward to its presence in my prayer life in the form of a purple light that guided me in many situations. I had often shared with my pastor about "my color purple," and he didn't recognize it as demonic either. Believing it was from the Lord, we were both deceived.

As a result of this demonic guide in the past year, my marriage has ended, my son is alienated from me, and I am alienated from my church.

Now as a result of an encounter with Truth, I am free in Christ. I truly know the peace that surpasses all understanding, and my heart and mind are guarded in Christ Jesus!

A Sound Mind

There is nothing wrong with visualizing or imagining doing certain things such as preaching a message in the power of the Holy Spirit. That is spiritually safe and potentially beneficial if two conditions are met. First, it should be for the benefit of something we plan to actually do. Peter wrote, "Gird your minds for action, keep sober in spirit, fix your hope completely on the grace to be brought to you at the revelation of Jesus Christ" (1 Pet. 1:13). Imagining yourself doing something or being someone without subsequent and appropriate action will lead to a departure from reality. One cannot distinguish over time something vividly and repeatedly imagined from what actually happened.

Second, what we visualize, or imagine, doing must conform to reality and be consistent with Scripture. Imagining, or visualizing, immoral acts will pollute the mind. Three viewings of hard-core pornography are said to have the same lasting impression on the mind as one actual experience. Paul wrote that "we have the mind of Christ" (1 Cor. 2:16) within us. Furthermore, Paul commands us to avoid losing control through intoxicating drink but, instead, to be filled with the Holy Spirit, implying that the Spirit should influence our thinking and behavior (see Eph. 5:18-19). The Holy Spirit is the Spirit of truth, and He will lead us into all truth, which will set us free (see John 8:32; 14:17; 16:13). We are to bring "into captivity every thought to the obedience of Christ" (2 Cor. 10:5, *KJV*). God holds us responsible for our own thoughts, and by His grace, we always have the capacity to choose what we are going to think or believe. Paul said, "God hath not given us the spirit of fear; but of power, and of love, and of a sound mind" (2 Tim. 1:7, *KJV*). The Greek word for "sound mind" is *sophronismos*, which is also translated "self-control" or "discipline." The Christian life is to be characterized by a self-disciplined mind.

Having the mind of Christ does not imply thought control by God, but rather, it is the ability to think like Christ because of His marvelous presence in our lives. However, we still have the responsibility to choose and examine our thoughts in the light of Scripture and Christ. If the thoughts are not true or consistent with His nature, then we shouldn't think or believe it. If our thoughts are not consistent with His, then we are to choose to believe His thoughts over ours. For example, suppose a Christian decided to believe that Jesus Christ is only one of many pathways to God. This idea directly conflicts with Jesus' statement in which He claimed, "I am the way, the truth, and the life; no man cometh unto the Father, but by me" (John 14:6, *KJV*). Therefore, by faith, we choose to believe what God says is true.

Our thinking should never come under the control of any other human being, regardless of who they are or who they claim to be. The apostle Paul praised the Bereans because, while they were eager to learn, they searched the

Scriptures daily to make sure that what he was saying was true (see Acts 17:11). History is filled with examples of people who failed to exercise this critical responsibility and suffered personal deception and devastation as a result. Remember the sad pictures of the hundreds who drank a poisoned drink under the order of cult-leader Jim Jones.

Paul summarizes how we should use our minds in Philippians 4:6-9:

> Be anxious for nothing, but in everything by prayer and supplication with thanksgiving let your requests be made known to God. And the peace of God, which surpasses all comprehension, shall guard your hearts and your minds in Christ Jesus. Finally, brethren, whatever is true, whatever is honorable, whatever is right, whatever is pure, whatever is lovely, whatever is of good repute, if there is any excellence and if anything worthy of praise, let your mind dwell on these things. The things you have learned and received and heard seen in me, practice these things; and the God of peace shall be with you.

Warning Signs

Biblical Christianity parts ways with much of the mind-body movement and is diametrically opposed to what New Age practitioners are teaching. In the latter, the individual typically attempts to do one of three things:

1. Empty the mind of all conscious thought in an attempt to become unified with a higher level of consciousness. This is the nature of transcendental meditation (TM).
2. Get in touch with one's inner self, subconscious or spirit.
3. Escape reality by imagining something that is not true (for example, picturing oneself in an environment in which he does not currently exist). In other words, the individual attempts to "trick" his body into believing what is not true.

In each case, the goal that is typically being sought is a state of relaxation or inner peace. But this is a cheap counterfeit for the peace and joy that only comes by the indwelling presence of God's Spirit within His children (see Gal. 5:22). Furthermore, the Holy Spirit never leaves the individual who abides in Christ (see John 15; Rom. 8:6; Gal. 5:22-25). Thirty minutes of visualization cannot make up for a day filled with wrong thought patterns and emotional responses.

> Thou wilt keep him in perfect peace, whose mind is stayed on thee: because he trusteth in thee (Isa. 26:3, *KJV*).

The problem for many Christians is that they fail to experience this kind of peace on a daily basis and, therefore, go searching for it through techniques such as described in this chapter. Why is this? The answer is because the truths of God's Word—which are necessary to bear the fruit of the Spirit—have either been forgotten or never known within the heart (see 2 Pet. 1:9). Others have never put into practice what they profess to believe. However, when these truths find agreement in a person's heart, the inevitable result is joy and peace.

> The statutes of the LORD are right, rejoicing the heart: the command-ment of the LORD is pure, enlightening the eyes (Ps. 19:8, *KJV*).

Benefits of Biblical Mind-Body Medicine

To experience the true benefits of mind-body medicine you need to do the following:

1. Resolve all known personal and spiritual conflicts through genuine repentance and faith in God. This is what the lady did, which she described in her letter. Central to this process is forgiving from the heart. Many psychosomatic illnesses are cured when bitterness is overcome by forgiveness.
2. "Let the peace of Christ rule in your hearts" (Col. 3:15). You do this by letting "the word of Christ dwell in you richly" (Col. 3:16). There is no substitute for knowing the Word of God. Other people cannot think or believe for you.
3. Meditate upon Scripture until your heart embraces the truth that will set you free. Meditation is not a New Age concept; it is a biblical discipline. Meditation will lead to spiritual bondage if it has the wrong focus (i.e., a mantra, an illusion, etc.). Biblical meditation involves "chewing the cud" of God's Word, spending time thinking

about its meaning, looking up cross-references and so on. "For to be carnally minded is death; but to be spiritually minded is life and peace" (Rom. 8:6, *KJV*).

4. Trust God and obey His Word. You can have the world's most powerful engine under your hood, but it does you no good until you engage the transmission. Obedience is faith in operation; it is like releasing the clutch on a manual transmission. A Bible-college professor used to say, "Impression without expression equals depression." As you live out what God shows you in the prayer closet, His truths take on even greater significance in your life.

5. Be filled with the Holy Spirit, and your life will manifest the fruit of the Spirit. Research demonstrates that when individuals experience positive emotional states, the physical heart demonstrates optimum electrical patterns that are not only beneficial to that key organ, but also influence the rest of the body. This is why "a sound heart is the life of the flesh" (Prov. 14:30, *KJV*), and why biblical mind-body medicine begins in a heart that is right with God.

Keep thy heart with all diligence; for out of it are the issues of life (Prov. 4:23, *KJV*).

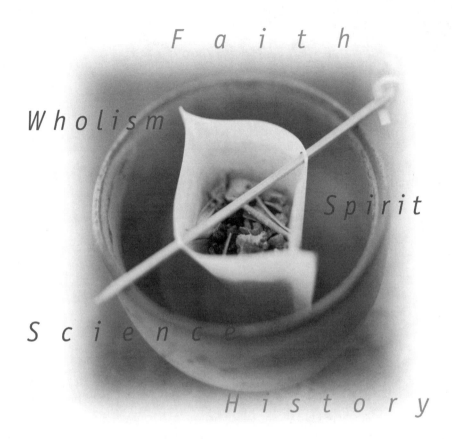

Faith

Wholism

Spirit

Science

History

PART 4

TO YOUR GOOD
HEALTH

CHAPTER TWENTY-ONE

A CHRISTIAN COMMITMENT TO WHOLISTIC HEALTH

Beloved, I pray that in all respects you may prosper and be in good health, just as your soul prospers.

3 JOHN 2

A young lady called and asked if she could have some personal time with me (Neil). She was willing to fly from the East Coast, where she lived, to meet with me in California, where I taught at Talbot School of Theology. She claimed to have deep spiritual, psychological and physical problems. And indeed, she did! She couldn't hide her disappointment with God, since she believed that He had promised her prosperity and good health. After hearing her story, I said, "You need to finish the verse you just quoted. Your prosperity and health are dependent upon how well your soul is doing. You have gone through rehabilitation three times for substance abuse. You have had two abortions and you have been married twice." I couldn't help but think that the verse was working.

We cannot violate the spiritual and natural laws that God has created and not expect some negative consequences. To enjoy life and experience good health requires us to take into account all of life's realities. God relates to His children as whole people and requires us to be good stewards of the life that He has entrusted to us. Therefore, we would like to conclude this book with some principles that we hope will guide you into making the right decisions concerning your physical, mental, emotional and spiritual health.

Principle #1: Seek First the Kingdom of God

Pray

The first thing a Christian should do about anything is pray. We have been conditioned to first seek every natural cause and remedy, but when that fails, there is nothing left to do but pray. However, Jesus said we should first seek His kingdom and then all the rest falls in line. Prayer works in conjunction with common sense. For example, if you fell from your roof and broke your leg, first pray and then call 911, or pray on your way to the nearest emergency room if you can get there. But no matter what—pray!

Whenever we get sick, the first thing we do is pray. We also pray for our children's sicknesses. At the first sign of illness, we need to lay our hands on them and pray. We ask for divine protection and wisdom. We ask the Lord to lay His healing hand on them and on ourselves. There is no promise that He will miraculously heal us, especially if we have violated His laws and have not assumed our own responsibility to eat and live right. However, James 4:2 says, "You do not have because you do not ask." In praying, we should desire nothing more or less than God's will. He may be allowing an illness for our spiritual good. Therefore, we pray:

> Lord, we submit ourselves to You and if it be Your will, we humbly ask You to heal our bodies of these illnesses. Show us where we have been negligent of our responsibility to live a wholesome life. If You are allowing this for a greater purpose, then enable us, by Your grace, to endure the suffering so that Your power may be perfected in our weakness.

Submit

We are urged by the mercies of God to submit our bodies to Him as living sacrifices (see Rom. 12:1). This has also become our first order of prayer. Whenever we sense cold or flu symptoms, we stop and pray, "Lord, I submit my body to You as a living sacrifice, and I ask You to fill me with Your Holy Spirit. I exercise the authority I have in Christ and command Satan and all his evil workers to leave my presence." According to James 4:7, we need to submit ourselves to God, but in order to take into account all reality, we also need to resist the devil, and he will flee from us. We can also call the elders and request prayer for our sickness. Calling the elders for prayer should always be done with the desire to be open and honest with God, and then be willing to confess and repent of any known sin.

In the spring of 1991, I (Neil) was suddenly overcome at school by what I thought to be a kidney-stone attack. I managed to make it to the emergency room at a local hospital where X rays revealed that I had four kidney stones. By the time the exam was over, the pain had subsided. I was given a prescription for pain medication and sent home.

That summer I went on a conference tour with four kidney stones embedded within me. On the Friday evenings before two conferences, I suddenly doubled over with pain. The natural tendency is to reach for the pain pills, but instead, I stopped and prayed, "Lord I give my body to you as a living sacrifice. I ask you to fill me with your Holy Spirit, and I command Satan in the name of Jesus to leave my presence." Miraculously, the pain stopped. Was it a natural coincidence? Could be. Was it a natural kidney-stone attack, and the Lord granted a partial healing in order that I could complete the conference? Could be. Was it a spiritual attack, and I just took authority over the enemy and the pain left? I personally think it was the latter, but I couldn't prove it to anyone; but I don't really have to. I simply did what Scripture told me to do, and so should every Christian.

That fall I had a lithotripsy procedure that used pulsating sound waves to break up the stones. It worked, and I passed them without further complications. How like Satan to attack under the disguise of a known physical condition. That is why we must be wholistic in our prayers and treatment.

PRINCIPLE #2: RESOLVE ALL PERSONAL AND SPIRITUAL CONFLICTS THROUGH GENUINE REPENTANCE AND FAITH IN GOD

Since most of the population is sick for psychosomatic reasons (i.e., illnesses due to stress, anxiety disorders, depression, anger, addictions, etc.), it is imperative that we have some means of resolving these conflicts. These illnesses not only affect us physically but also spiritually. We need to have a regular spiritual check-up, and that is probably why God initiated the ordinance of Communion. Paul instructed the Church in 1 Corinthians 11:28-30 to partake in Communion in order to stay spiritually healthy.

But let a man examine himself, and so let him eat of the bread and drink of the cup. For he who eats and drinks, eats and drinks judgment to himself, if he does not judge the body rightly. For this reason many among you are weak and sick, and a number sleep.

Independent research is being conducted on the approach that Freedom in Christ Ministries uses to resolve personal and spiritual conflicts. The research was conducted on those who requested a personal appointment. Each was given one extensive counseling session (three to five hours), where a lay encourager took them through the Steps to Freedom in Christ. The results (after one conference) are as follows:

57 percent improved in depression
54 percent improved in anxiety
49 percent improved in fear
55 percent improved in anger
50 percent improved in tormenting or disturbing thoughts
53 percent improved in negative habits
56 percent improved in self-esteem[1]

These high results cannot help but improve the quality of life and significantly reduce psychosomatic illnesses. Such fruit is only possible when the pastoral counselors take into account the reality of the spiritual world and understand that Jesus is the wonderful counselor. Whenever a Christian doctor, pastor or counselor ministers to another individual, God is there. And there is a role that only He can play in the life of His children. Only Jesus can forgive our sins, give us life, bind up the brokenhearted and set the captives free.

We understand that some conflicts cannot be resolved in a short time because of the complex nature of the client's difficulties. We also know that resolution will necessitate a change in lifestyle, and that also takes time. To maintain our freedom in Christ we must learn how to forgive from our hearts, find our hope in God, cast all our anxieties upon Him and overcome the temptations of this world. This means that we need to learn how to live by faith according to what God says is true in the power of the Holy Spirit.

PRINCIPLE #3: LIVE A BALANCED LIFE OF REST, EXERCISE AND DIET (RED)

Rest

God established the seven-day week and instructed us to take one day of rest. Our bodies need to have some time to recover from six days of labor. The average person also needs seven to eight hours of sleep each night. You can burn the candle at both ends for a while, but eventually it will catch up with you.

There is another kind of rest, however, that is even more important for your overall health. Jesus said, "Come to Me, all who are weary and heavy-laden, and I will give you rest" (Matt. 11:28). He is not talking about the cessation of labor or an abdication of personal responsibility. He is talking about living our lives by faith in His power. If we try to serve God in our own strength and resources, we will burn out. The stresses generated by our own self-centered living will consume us. We don't naturally live our lives for God. The supernatural life of Christ is lived out through us by faith.

> Physical health begins with good mental health, and mentally healthy people are those who have a right relationship with the Lord.

Physical and spiritual disciplines are necessary for wholistic health. The Lord has asked us to give Him the first hour of the day, the first day of the week and the first of our income. The firstfruits are what he takes and multiplies, not what is left over at the end of the day. Physical health begins with good mental health, and mentally healthy people are those who have a right relationship with their creator. If you knew that God loved you, that your sins were forgiven, that He had prepared a place for you for all eternity, that sin and physical death no longer had any power over you and that your life was characterized by the fruit of the Spirit, would you be a mentally healthy person? Would you feel good about yourself? Of course you would, and every child of God has the same privileges and the same opportunity to be the person God created him or her to be.

Exercise

For your physical health, aerobic exercises are the best for your cardiovascular system. The idea is to have some sustained exercise for 20 to 30 minutes.

It should be strenuous enough to increase your heart rate from 120 to 150 beats per minute, depending on your age. After 15 to 20 minutes, you should feel flush, which is indicative that your blood is reaching the capillaries in your extremities. You can accomplish this by running, jogging, brisk walking, biking, swimming or some other kind of aerobic exercise three or four times a week.

Diet

For proper diet, we recommend that you read Michael's book *The Word on Health* (which is also designed to build a proper doctrinal framework for wholistic health) and *What the Bible Says About Healthy Living* by Rex Russell. Most of us have some reasonable idea of what constitutes healthy food. Making a commitment to follow it is the difficult part. We have observed that law-based programs don't work. We are under a new covenant of grace, and we must learn to live by faith in the power of the Holy Spirit. *The Diet Alternative* by Diane Hampton (Whitaker House, 2002) is one of the few books on the market that talks about eating food from a grace perspective.

Finding the proper rest, exercise and diet is a question of biblical balance. We are to do all things in moderation. If we focus too much on one thing, we take our eyes off the Lord. Balance comes when we live under the grace of God by faith.

PRINCIPLE #4: DON'T SACRIFICE YOUR ETERNAL SOUL FOR TEMPORAL GAINS

Counterfeit religious systems will probably gain more access to the Church through medicine in the coming years than any other way. Jesus said:

> For what will a man be profited, if he gains the whole world, and forfeits his soul? Or what will a man give in exchange for his soul? (Matt. 16:26).

Christians will be tempted to submit to almost any treatment in order get pain relief or to effect a cure. This is essentially the same temptation that affects chemically addicted people every day—they start using in order to stop the pain or to cope with life. The results are disastrous in the long run. Some of the most lucrative industries in America are those that peddle temporary relief from anxiety and pain.

If you have been reading this book carefully, then you should know what to do before you submit to any treatment plan. First, check the history of the founder or product and treatment plan. Read the label and ask for the literature that supports the products or advice. Second, find out the operating faith behind the procedure or product. Third, consider a wholistic answer. Are you dealing with the symptoms or the root causes? Fourth, see if the product or procedure agrees with natural law (science). Is there any research to back up the product, advice or procedure? Fifth, determine if the spiritual realm is involved, and if so, is it the Holy Spirit or another spirit? Finally, do you have a peace about it? Is the Holy Spirit leading you, or do you sense a different spirit?

Many Americans believe that pain is an intolerable enemy that must be eradicated. That is not true. If we couldn't feel pain, we would be a hopeless mask of scars within a matter of days and weeks. We suggest you read *Pain: The Gift Nobody Wants* by Dr. Paul Brand and Philip Yancey. Learning to live with pain is an important part of the growth process. However, there is no value in suffering needlessly if there are proper means to reduce the pain without impairing judgment.

Pain and suffering are part of the sanctifying process. The old athletic adage, No pain, no gain, also applies to the spiritual realm. There is no painless way to die to self-rule.

> For we who live are constantly being delivered over to death for Jesus' sake, that the life of Jesus also may be manifested in our mortal flesh (2 Cor. 4:11).

PRINCIPLE #5: SEEK THE OPINIONS AND PERSPECTIVES OF OTHERS

> Where there is no guidance, the people fall, but in abundance of counselors there is victory (Prov. 11:14).

There are no perfect doctors, counselors or pastors. No one person has the perfect perspective and all the answers. If your doctor is recommending a major surgery that you do not have peace about, seek a second opinion. It is your life, not his or hers, and ultimately, it is your responsibility. In order to be a good steward of the life that God has entrusted you (see 1 Cor. 4:1-5), you need to seek the perspective of others. No one discipline has the total perspective either. Your pastor does not know what your doctor does, and generally speaking, neither one has been schooled in good nutrition.

Wholistic health requires the input of many disciplines. For instance, allopathic cancer treatment centers have traditionally brought the oncologist, surgeon and radiologist together to determine the proper treatment. They will discuss whether they should kill the bad cells with chemicals or radiation, or whether they should cut the cancerous cells out. One has to wonder if doctors and scientists 100 years from now will look at these destructive and invasive practices as barbaric? Can cancer be prevented with a proper balance of rest, exercise and diet? Can heart disease? Can diabetes? Should the treatment for cancer, heart disease and diabetes be more wholistic? We think it should, and we believe that the Christian community should be taking the lead in wholistic medicine. Wisdom is seeing life from God's perspective. May He enable you to make the right choices for your health as you seek Him with all your heart.

THE MOST CRITICAL STEP TO BIBLICAL WHOLISTIC HEALTH

This is a book that discusses alternative medicines from a biblical standpoint. In it, we present a paradigm that acknowledges all three dimensions of our being—spirit, soul and body. Optimum health flows from proper care of all three aspects of our whole person. Therefore, we would be remiss if we did not at least introduce the biblical process for achieving healthiness and wholeness.

According to the Bible, every human being is born spiritually dead, that is, separated from God. Paul wrote:

> Through one man [Adam] sin entered the world, and death through sin, and thus death spread to all men, because all sinned (Rom. 5:12, *NKJV*).

Physical death is also a consequence of the Fall, but for Adam that came many hundreds of years later. As a result of the Fall, we are all prone to sickness and eventually physical death.

HOW CAN WE BE SPIRITUALLY ALIVE?

This was essentially the question posed by the Jewish ruler Nicodemus to Jesus Christ, who answered by saying:

> Unless one is born of water and the Spirit, he cannot enter into the kingdom of God. That which is born of the flesh is flesh, and that which is born of the Spirit is spirit (John 3:5-6, *NKJV*).

In other words, just as your current physical existence required that you be born once, your spirit also must be born. This rebirth cannot come about by any human initiative or means, such as doing good works, giving money to the poor, attending church or anything else. Instead, it can only come about as a result of God, the heavenly Father, placing His Spirit within our hearts.

HOW IS ONE BORN AGAIN BY THE SPIRIT?

Jesus said, "For God so loved the world that He gave His only begotten Son, that whoever believes in Him should not perish but have everlasting life" (John 3:16, *NKJV*). Being born again comes about by faith—a change in belief—so that your confidence and trust are no longer in yourself (or what you can do) to have a relationship with God. Instead, you put your confidence and trust in the sacrificial death and resurrection of God's perfect, sinless Son, Jesus Christ, whose death paid the penalty for your sin. You can have an exclusive relationship with God when you put your trust in what Jesus did on the cross for each and every one of His children.

> For the wages [due compensation] of sin is death, but the gift of God is eternal life in Christ Jesus our Lord (Rom. 6:23, *NKJV*).

Isaiah the prophet predicted that Jesus, the Messiah, as a sacrificial lamb, would take the penalty for our sin upon Himself.

> But He was wounded for our transgressions, He was bruised for our iniquities; the chastisement for our peace was upon Him, and by His stripes we are healed (Isa. 53:5, *NKJV*).

This accomplished the rebirth of the spirit. "For as in Adam all die, even so in Christ all shall be made alive" (1 Cor. 15:22, *NKJV*).

Jesus said:

I am the way, the truth, and the life. No one comes to the Father except through Me (John 14:6, *NKJV*).

Peter affirmed this when he said, "Nor is there salvation in any other, for there is no other name under heaven given among men by which we must be saved" (Acts 4:12, *NKJV*).

In stating this, we should also point out two things.

1. Every faith/religion claims to articulate the right path to truth and immortality. In other words, each religion proclaims its own opinion as to how one can be made whole. As such, each religion is by nature exclusive of the others.
2. Every individual is a person of faith. Even an atheist is a person of faith. The reason for this is that faith refers to what you believe and who you believe. All of us believe something about the big questions of life, and each of us has chosen to believe someone's answers to those questions. So, with regard to faith, the question is not, Do you believe (something)? but rather, Who have you chosen to believe? and, Are they worthy of your trust (faith)?

We believe that there is no one more worthy of our trust than Jesus Christ. He showed us perfect wholeness and a right relationship with God the Father, and He gave His life for us so that we might have the privilege to be made whole. Furthermore, we believe that there is no book on Earth more worthy of our trust than the Bible, which documents Jesus' story and provides the only legitimate answer to man's predicament in his pursuit of wholistic health—the means to a regenerated spirit and a restored relationship with his creator.

The Bible reveals to us that, through faith in Christ, we once again have the incredible opportunity to be made whole by becoming children of God.

But as many as received him, to them gave he power to become the sons of God, even to them that believe on his name: which were born, not of blood, nor of the will of the flesh, nor of the will of man, but of God (John 1:12-13, *KJV*).

WHY NOT TRUST IN GOD TODAY?

We are grateful for the good physical life and health that God has given to us. But far more precious to us than our bodies, which even now are in the process of decay and inevitable death, is the new and eternal life we share through Jesus Christ as sons of God. If you have never responded from your heart to God's priceless invitation to be born of His Spirit through faith in Jesus Christ, won't you do so now?

Dear Lord Jesus,
I acknowledge that I am a sinner and need Your forgiveness in this fallen
world. I believe that You died for my sins on the cross of Calvary, and I desire to
turn from my sin and my wicked ways. Please come into my life and create in
me a clean heart and a new and right spirit. As You gave Your life for me,
so I now give my life back to You. I receive You today as my Lord and Savior.
In Jesus' name, amen.

For whosoever shall call upon the name of the Lord shall be saved (Rom. 10:13, *KJV*).

If you just took this critical step to wholeness, we congratulate you and welcome you as a brother or sister in Christ. Because a newborn cannot survive on his own without daily food and a nurturing parent, we suggest that you begin to feed yourself spiritually by reading the Bible (beginning with the Gospel of John) daily and by joining a good Bible-teaching church in your area.

WHERE ARE THE HEALING MIRACLES TODAY?

Because of the relative obscurity of supernatural healing during the majority of the Church's history, many Christians have concluded that the supernatural gift of healing diminished with the apostles and is no longer in existence, or it is reserved for special purposes as determined only by God. Evidence cited to support this premise are several Scriptures that indicate that the primary purpose for these healing miracles was to prove the deity of Christ and to validate the gospel message.

> But that ye may know that the Son of man hath power on earth to forgive sins, (then saith he to the sick of the palsy,) arise, take up thy bed, and go unto thine house (Matt. 9:6, *KJV*).

> And when he had called unto him his twelve disciples, he gave them power against unclean spirits, to cast them out, and to heal all manner of sickness and all manner of disease. And as ye go, preach, saying, the kingdom of heaven is at hand. Heal the sick, cleanse the lepers, raise the dead (Matt. 10:1,7-8, *KJV*).

> How shall we escape, if we neglect so great salvation; which at the first began to be spoken by the Lord, and was confirmed unto us by them that heard him; God also bearing them witness, both with signs and wonders, and with divers miracles, and gifts of the Holy Ghost, according to his own will? (Heb. 2:3-4, *KJV*).

It goes without saying that God has not lost his power to heal. Furthermore, there is no question that miracles of healing still occur. Not only have we witnessed God's touch on His children, but other reported miracles are not uncommon. This especially seems to be the case in areas where the gospel is just being introduced or revival is taking place.

Should we expect then that once evangelization has occurred God will suspend the gift of healing? Or are there other reasons why the gift of healing is not as prominent? Believing that God always has the power to heal, we need to consider some possible reasons why we are not seeing this miraculous intervention more in our church communities.

WE ARE CALLED TO SEEK THE GIVER AND NOT THE GIFT

Although gifts play an important role in the life of the Church, it is the Lord Himself whom we are to seek. As we yield ourselves to Him, He distributes gifts to every individual just as He wills (see 1 Cor. 12:11). It is legitimate to earnestly desire that the believers in Christ receive gifts so that the whole Church is edified, but it is not legitimate to desire gifts to make us individually more prominent. Paul wrote, "If there are gifts of prophecy, they will be done away; if there are tongues, they will cease; if there is knowledge, it will be done away. For we know in part, and we prophesy in part; but when the perfect comes, the partial will be done away" (1 Cor. 13:8-10). In other words, gifts come and go, but what remains is faith, hope and love (see 1 Cor. 13:13). During this Church age, God will give gifts as He sees fit for the edification of the Church and for the need of the moment. The constant that we are to strive for is faith, hope and love.

We have witnessed God's miraculous healings on several occasions, although not consistently through one specific method or individual. God seems to sovereignly touch some and not others. Sometimes God responds to our prayers of faith, and other times He chooses to heal those who showed no faith or desire to be healed (see John 5:1-16). While we don't know why He chooses to miraculously intervene in some and not others, we do know that His Word is sure, and if we live by faith according to what He says is true, we will live better, healthier, longer lives and bear more fruit.

Some have argued that God can only be glorified when a Christian is healed, and that is the only way we can be a positive witness to the unbelieving medical field. That is not true. Nurses and doctors may turn to God when they witness a miraculous healing, but they are turned off to God when they see Christians respond poorly to illness or the loss of a loved one. What causes unbelievers to sit up and take notice is when the faith of Christians is proved as they endure their suffering with joy and patience. Calmly accepting the death of loved ones—knowing that they are in the presence of God—and graciously accepting God's will even when it involves suffering and loss is what we as believers need to show the world. Although Paul brought healing to many, the Lord never answered His prayer that a thorn be removed from his own flesh. God allowed it to keep Paul humble. In this way the Lord will use sickness and suffering to build our character. For power is perfected in weakness, and God will do whatever is necessary in order to keep us from exalting ourselves (see 2 Cor. 12:9).

Historians have noticed what tends to happen to faith healers of other religions. In ancient Greece, the sick went to doctor-priests who practiced their art at local Greek temples. Perhaps due to pressure to produce results, these healers often resorted to fraud as a substitute for supernatural intervention.[1] Unfortunately, this type of deception has not been absent from the cadre of faith healers in Christian circles today. A television evangelist-healer utilized an earpiece that received transmissions from a staff member who was parked in a nearby van. The staff member collected information cards on people in the audience and then verbalized their contents to the healer via the earpiece. Exposure of such fraud has been an embarrassment to the Truth that such Christian healers claim to represent. We are not saying that God could not give the gift of healing to an individual, but we are saying that the focus should be on Christ and the need of the sick, not on the minister. We are also saying that the message of the Church is never one dimensional, and whatever is taught and practiced must be consistent with the whole message of the Bible.

WE ARE CALLED TO FOCUS ON THE ETERNAL AND SPIRITUAL VERSUS THE TEMPORAL AND NATURAL

While Jesus did feed the 5,000, restored sight to the blind and hearing to the deaf, many times he instructed those He healed not to tell others. If the only purpose for His miracles was to verify His ministry, then why would He ask them not to tell others? Because physical healing was not His purpose for coming to Earth. He came to meet our eternal and spiritual needs by dying on the cross for our sins and then resurrecting in order that we may have eternal life in Christ. In fact, He knew that if He healed the sick and fed the 5,000, that would be the primary reason people came to see Him. It is the fickle nature of humanity to focus on temporal and physical needs while overlooking our eternal and spiritual needs, which is probably why Jesus asked those He healed not to share how they were healed with others. So why did He do it? Because it was His nature to do it. Throughout the Gospels we read that Jesus was moved by compassion when He saw the needs of a suffering humanity, and He still is moved today. For that we are eternally grateful.

WE ARE CALLED TO FOCUS ON OBEDIENCE, NOT THE MIRACULOUS

The reason for this should be obvious—God created the fixed order of the universe and the physical laws of nature. It is false to conclude that God is only involved when He works outside the established order He created. For example, if we violate what God's Word states and find ourselves physically impaired, it is likely that God allowed us to experience the natural consequences of our choices. Consider the analogy of someone who poured water into their gas tank. They would have no one to blame but themselves for the adverse consequences that would surely follow. Likewise, we can't eat with reckless abandon and then expect God to heal us when we get sick. If that were the case, we would all violate our temples (bodies) all week, confess it on the weekend—expecting God to eradicate the consequences of our sinful choices—and then repeat the same behavior the following week. Thank God we don't have to live with the eternal consequences of our sins, but we do have to live with many of the temporal consequences. It is a far greater miracle to see God's will accomplished through the Church and His established order in spite of the fact that not one of us is perfectly trustworthy.

WE ARE CALLED TO CAST OUT DEMONS, NOT DISEASES

When the Lord was training the twelve disciples, He "gave them power and authority over all demons, and to cure diseases" (Luke 9:1, *NKJV*). The spiritual authority that every believer has in Christ is over the kingdom of darkness (i.e., Satan and his demons). Demons are personal beings, but diseases are not. By the authority and power we have in Christ, and by the name of Jesus, we can command Satan and his demons to depart from us, but we can't command germs and viruses in the natural realm to leave. Jesus is our immune system in the spiritual realm, but living a balanced life of rest, exercise and diet, according to Scripture, is what strengthens our immune system in the natural realm. For the former, see Neil's book *The Bondage Breaker* (Harvest House, 1994), and for the latter, see Michael's book *The Word on Health* (Moody Press, 2000).

WE ARE CALLED TO SALVATION

The psalmist wrote, "Who [God] pardons all your iniquities; who heals all your diseases" (Ps. 103:3; see also Exod. 15:26; Jer. 30:17). Such passages have led some to believe that the atoning work of Christ not only saved us from our sins, but also healed all our diseases. This is true from an eternal perspective. Every child of God is forgiven and is now in the process of conforming to His image. However, both salvation and sanctification as applied to the believer are presented in past, present and future tense. In other words, we have been saved (see Titus 3:4-5), we are being saved (see 1 Cor. 1:18), and some day we will be fully saved from the wrath that is to come (see Rom. 5:9-10). In the same way, we have been sanctified (see 1 Cor. 6:11), we are being sanctified (see Rom. 6:22), and some day we shall be fully sanctified (see 1 Thess. 3:12-13).

We have not yet experienced the totality of either our salvation or our sanctification. We can, however, be assured of our salvation. "These things I have written to you who believe in the name of the Son of God, in order that you may know that you have eternal life" (1 John 5:13). And we have been "sealed in Him [Christ] with the Holy Spirit of promise, who is given as a pledge of our inheritance" (Eph. 1:13-14). We will not experience complete healing until we receive our resurrected bodies and are in the presence of the Lord in eternity. Until then we will continue living in dying bodies in this fallen world. We cannot claim by faith that we be fully healed any more than we can claim by faith that we have resurrected bodies and that we are perfectly sanctified. We can and should claim by faith what God says is true and then seek to live accordingly.

WE ARE CALLED TO FELLOWSHIP WITH THE HOLY SPIRIT

Gifts of healing are gifts of the Spirit. They come from God, as does the fruit of the Spirit. The Holy Spirit is one of three Persons with whom we as Christians have a personal relationship and with whom we are to continually walk in fellowship (see Gal. 5:16). But we can cut ourselves off from fellowship with the Spirit. While out of fellowship with Him, we will not experience His blessings, because they are a manifestation of His life in us. Such physical, mental, emotional and spiritual blessings are a direct by-product of our relationship with Him. It is like unplugging a lamp from the outlet; no light can be emitted when it is cut off from its power source. Jesus said, "Abide in me . . . for without me ye can do *nothing*" (John 15:4-5, *KJV*, emphasis added).

We Grieve the Holy Spirit When We Fail to Love Others

Jesus left this earth so that He could indwell us by the Holy Spirit (see John 16:7). As a result, He now lives in us and desires to communicate His love to others through us. We are to openly channel His love to others. Prior to Paul's command to walk in fellowship with the Holy Spirit, he tells us "all the law is fulfilled in one word, even in this; Thou shalt love thy neighbor as thyself" (Gal. 5:14, *KJV*). Jesus said that if we come to God and remember that our brother has something against us, we should go and first be reconciled to our brother and then return to Him (see Matt. 5:23-24). We cannot have fellowship with God while having enmity with another human being. John said it this way, "If a man say, I love God, and hateth his brother, he is a liar: for he that loveth not his brother whom he hath seen, how can he love God whom he hath not seen?" (1 John 4:20, *KJV*).

Peter exhorted husbands to honor their wives and live with them in wisdom and understanding so "that your prayers be not hindered" (1 Pet. 3:7, *KJV*). Jesus also taught us to ask God to forgive us for our debts in accordance with how we forgive others (see Matt. 6:12). He also warned us that if we don't forgive others from the heart, we will be turned over to the tormentors (see Matt. 18:34-35). Such bitterness is a major cause of spiritual bondage and psychosomatic illness. Instead of experiencing the joy of salvation and the fruit of the Holy Spirit, the lives of bitter people are characterized by mental torment, fear, anxiety, insomnia, depression and anger.

We Grieve the Holy Spirit When We Yield Our Bodies to Sin

Grieving the Holy Spirit occurs when we use our bodies as instruments of unrighteousness and allow sin to reign in our mortal bodies (see Rom. 6:11-13). You can't commit a sexual sin without using your body as an instrument of unrighteousness. Therefore, if you have committed a sexual sin, you have allowed sin to reign in your mortal body. You will not only be in spiritual bondage, but also you will be in danger of suffering physically from sexually transmitted diseases (STDs) and other abnormalities. As Christians, we can live according to the Spirit or we can live according to the flesh (see Gal. 5:19-23). The deeds of the flesh include immorality, anger, strife, hatred, discord, jealousy, envy, drunkenness and a lack of self-control. Such attitudes and behaviors are another cause of many psychosomatic illnesses.

We Grieve the Holy Spirit When We Practice Iniquity

Iniquity is a slightly different concept from sin. The Greek word for "sin" is *hamartia*. At the time of Christ, hamartia was used as an archery term, referring to someone's failure to hit the bull's-eye. Hamartia presupposes that the archer was doing his best to nail the bull's-eye but still failed. In other words, even when we do our best, we fall short of God's standard of perfection and, therefore, we sin. Iniquity is when we are self-willed. It is being self-centered, self-sufficient and self-reliant. In the archery analogy, someone living in iniquity could not care if they hit the bull's-eye. They disregard the target and shoot somewhere else. King David said, "If I regard iniquity in my heart, the Lord will not hear me" (Ps. 66:18, *KJV*). Iniquity grieves the heart of God.

We Grieve the Holy Spirit When We Don't Trust Him

The words "faith," "believe" and "trust" in Scripture are all translated from the same Greek word. When you believe in someone, you are putting your trust in him or her. Faith is a demonstrated reliance in someone or something; it is not just a mental ascent. If we truly believe, faith will affect our walk and our talk. Faith was often a critical factor in whether or not Jesus healed someone from their malady. Jesus said it was faith that healed the woman with a hemorrhage, a blind man, a leper, and it was faith that raised Jairus's daughter from the dead (see Mark 5:25-42; 10:52; Luke 17:15-19). Even in Jesus' hometown, He "did not do many miracles there because of their unbelief" (Matt. 13:58). Paul healed the paralytic once he perceived that this man who had never walked "had faith to be healed" (Acts 14:9, *KJV*).

However, it is spiritually abusive to tell sick Christians that if they only had enough faith, they would be healed. This concept presupposes that it is God's will that everyone be healed. As we saw in chapter 4, that is not a biblically valid assumption. There is a difference between faith and presumption. Faith is based upon God's decree. If God has said He will heal everyone, then He will, and the individual has the choice to believe Him. However, God has not said that He will heal everyone—to believe that He will is presumption. Faith must be based in the absolute truth of God's Word, not on our own earthly thoughts and ideas.

We Grieve the Holy Spirit When We Strive for Perfection Under the Law

Paul asked: Did you receive the Spirit by the works of the law or by hearing with faith? Are you so foolish? Having begun by the Spirit, are you now perfected by the flesh? So then, does He who provides you with the Spirit and works miracles among you do it by the works of the law or by hearing with faith? (see Gal. 3:5). We are saved and sanctified by faith. Legalism and perfectionism lead only to stress, which is the cause for all kinds of illnesses. When we strive to secure God's approval on the basis of our own merits, we place ourselves back under the law and the curse it carries to those who fail to achieve its standard of perfection (see Gal. 3:10-11). You cannot earn good standing with God, because you already have it. By faith you are alive and free in Christ. Watchman Nee put it this way, "Oh, it is a great thing to see that we are in Christ! Think of the bewilderment of trying to get into a room in which you already are! Think of the absurdity of asking to be put in! If we recognize the fact that we are in, we make no effort to enter."[2]

The blessedness of being a child of God became yours the day you affirmed that Jesus Christ is the Son of God, and that the blood He shed on the cross of Calvary paid for all your sins. "He that spared not his own Son, but delivered him up for us all, how shall he not with him also freely give us all things?" (Rom. 8:32). In other words, don't grieve the Spirit by transferring your trust from Him to yourself. You don't have to, but more important, you can't earn God's unconditional love and acceptance. You already have it in Christ.

1. Brian Inglis, *A History of Medicine* (Cleveland, OH: The World Publishing Company, 1965), pp. 23-24.
2. Watchman Nee, *The Normal Christian Life* (Wheaton, IL: Tyndale House Publishers, 1977), n.p.

SCIENTIFIC RESEARCH RESULTS

TABLE B-1   HOMEOPATHY—CLINICAL TRIALS

Year	Author	No.	Remedy	Clinical Problem	Help?
1983	Shipley[1]		*Rhus toxicodendron* 6X	Osteoarthritis	No
1989	Fisher[2]	30	*Rhus toxicodendron* 6c	Fibrositis	Yes
1994	de Lange de Klerk[3]	175	Various	Upper respiratory infections in children	No
1995	Lokken[4]	24	Various (6)	(1) Postoperative pain (2) inflammation after wisdom tooth extraction	No
1995	Wiesenauer[5]	164	*Galphimia glauca*	Hay fever (study ended after 2 follow-up visits)	Yes
1996	Kainz[6]	60	Various	Warts	No
1997	Whitmarsh[7]	60	Various	Migraine headache	No
1998	Smolle[8]	60	Various	Warts	No
1999	Adler[9]	119	Sinusitis PMD® (*Lobaria pulmonaria, Luffa operculata,* Potassium dichromate)	Acute sinusitis (This was an "open-label" study. In other words, it was not blinded nor was it placebo-controlled to remove bias.)	Yes
2001	Walach[10]	18	Various	Headaches (This was a 1 yr. follow-up from a previous double-blind study.)	No
2001	Fisher[11]	112	Various	Rheumatoid arthritis	No

CONTINUED ON NEXT PAGE

TABLE B-1 CONTINUED

[1] M. Shipley et al., "Controlled Trial of Homoeopathic Treatment of Osteoarthritis," *Lancet* 1, no. 8316 (1983): 97-8.

[2] P. Fisher et al., "Effect of Homeopathic Treatment on Fibrositis (Primary Fibromyalgia)," *Brit Med J* 299, no. 6695 (1989): 365-6.

[3] E. S. de Lange de Klerk et al., "Effect of Homoeopathic Medicines on Daily Burden of Symptoms in Children with Recurrent Upper Respiratory Tract Infections," *Brit Med J* 309, no. 6965 (1994): 1329-32.

[4] Per Lokken et al., "Effect of Homeopathy on Pain and Other Events After Acute Trauma: Placebo-Controlled Trial with Bilateral Oral Surgery," *Brit Med J* 310 (1995): 1439-42.

[5] M. Wiesenauer and R. Ludtke, "The Treatment of Pollinosis with Galphimia Glauca D4: A Randomized Placebo-Controlled Double-Blind Clinical Trial," *Phytomedicine* 2, no. 1 (1995): 3-6.

[6] J. T. Kainz et al., "Homeopathic Versus Placebo Therapy of Children with Warts on the Hands: A Randomized, Double-Blind Clinical Trial," *Dermatology* 193, no. 4 (1996): 318-20.

[7] T. E. Whitmarsh, D. M. Coleston-Shields, and T. J. Steiner, "Double-Blind Randomized Placebo-Controlled Study of Homeopathic Prophylaxis of Migraine," *Cephalalgia* 17, no. 5 (1997): 600-4.

[8] J. Smolle, G. Prause, and H. Kerl, "A Double-Blind, Controlled Clinical Trial of Homeopathy and an Analysis of Lunar Phases and Postoperative Outcome," *Arch Dermatol* 134, no. 11 (1998): 1368-70.

[9] M. Adler, "Efficacy and Safety of a Fixed-Combination Homeopathic Therapy for Sinusitis," *Adv Ther* 16, no. 2 (1999): 103-11.

[10] H. Walach et al., "The Long-Term Effects of Homeopathic Treatment of Chronic Headaches: One Year Follow-Up and Single Case Time Series Analysis," *Brit Homeopathic J* 90, no. 2 (2001): 63-72.

[11] P. Fisher and D. L. Scott, "A Randomized Controlled Trial of Homeopathy in Rheumatoid Arthritis," *Rheumatology (Oxford)* 40, no. 9 (2001): 1052-5.

TABLE B-2   ACUPUNCTURE—CLINICAL TRIALS

Year	Author	No.	Clinical Problem	Nature of Study	Help?
1994	Molsberger,[1] Germany	48	Tennis elbow pain	Single-blind v. sham needling Only looked at immediate pain relief Acupuncture gave 20 hrs. relief; sham needle 1.4	Yes
1997	Appiah,[2] Germany	33	Raynaud's syndrome	Randomized controlled trial Received 7 acupuncture treatments Control group: no treatment Acupuncture group had less attacks + improved in capillary flow	Yes

CONTINUED ON NEXT PAGE

TABLE B-2 CONTINUED

Year	Author	No.	Clinical Problem	Nature of Study	Help?
1997	Jerner,[3] Sweden	56	Psoriasis	Single-blind (electrostimulation of acupuncture needles v. sham needling) 2x/wk. for 10 wks. Followed up 3 mos. after therapy	No
1997	Clavel-Chapelon,[4] France	996	Smoking cessation	The study looked at success of smoking cessation 4 yrs. after attempts to quit 4 groups: (1) nicotine gum + acupuncture (2) double placebo (3) gum + sham acupuncture (4) placebo gum + acupuncture	No
1997	Abuaisha,[5] England		Diabetic neuropathy (disease of nerves in legs from diabetes)	Nonrandomized; no placebo ≤6 acupuncture treatments over 10 wks. Follow-up from 18 to 52 wks. Reduction in symptoms and medication	Yes
1998	David,[6] England	70	Neck pain	Randomized study Acupuncture v. physical therapy Treatment for 6 wks. Followed up at 6 mos.	Same as physical therapy
1999	Jensen,[7] Norway	75	Patellofemoral pain (knee cap)	Randomized study Acupuncture 2x/wk. for 4 wks. v. no treatment Followed up for 1 yr.	Yes
1999	Mazzoni,[8] Italy	40	Obesity	Randomized; placebo-controlled 12 sessions of acupuncture v. moxibustion-acupuncture v. ear acupuncture Measured body mass, eating attitudes, anxiety, depression and quality of life 18 of 40 dropped out (6 of acupuncture, 12 control)	No

CONTINUED ON NEXT PAGE

TABLE B-2 CONTINUED

Year	Author	No.	Clinical Problem	Nature of Study	Help?
2000	Park,[9] England		Tinnitus (ringing in the ears)	This paper summarized the results of 6 available controlled trials on tinnitus and acupuncture	No*
2000	Honjo,[10] Japan	13	Urinary incontinence due to spinal cord injuries	Acupuncture given weekly for 4 wks. into skin of 3rd sacral foramina (holes)	Yes**
				Incontinence resolved in 2 (15%) and decreased to ≤50% in another 6 (46%)	
				Bladder capacity improved as well	
2000	Roschke,[11] Germany	70	Major depression	Single-blind; placebo-controlled	No
				All patients on an antidepressant drug	
				Acupuncture v. sham acupuncture v. none	
				Sham acupuncture did slightly better than rest	
2000	White,[12] England	50	Tension headache	Multicenter randomized controlled trial	No
				Acupuncture v. sham needling	
				Follow up for 3 mos.	
2000	Karst,[13] Germany	39	Tension headache	Double-blind placebo-controlled	No
				Acupuncture v. placebo acupuncture	
2000	Margolin,[14] USA	620	Cocaine addiction	Multicenter randomized single-blind	No
				12 different clinics and centers	
				Ear acupuncture v. sham needle v. relaxation	
				5 treatments/wk. for 8 wks. with drug counseling	
				Follow up at 3 and 6 mos.	
2000	White,[15] England		Smoking cessation	Review of randomized trials in literature	No
				20 studies comparing acupuncture v. sham acupuncture v. other interventions v. no intervention	

CONTINUED ON NEXT PAGE

TABLE B-2 CONTINUED

*2 unblinded studies showed acupuncture helped, but 4 blinded studies showed it of no benefit

**Nonrandomized; no controls

[1] A. Molsberger and E. Hille, "The Analgesic Effect of Acupuncture in Chronic Tennis Elbow Pain," *Brit J Rheumatol* 33, no. 12 (1994): 1162-5.

[2] R. Appiah et al., "Treatment of Primary Raynaud's Syndrome with Traditional Chinese Acupuncture," *J Intern Med* 241, no. 2 (1997): 119-24.

[3] B. Jerner, M. Skogh, and A. Vahlquist, "A Controlled Trial of Acupuncture in Psoriasis: No Convincing Effect," *Acta Derm-Venereol (Stockholm)* 77, no. 2 (1997): 154-6.

[4] F. Clavel-Chapelon, C. Paoletti, and S. Benhamou, "Smoking Cessation Rates 4 Years After Treatment by Nicotine Gum and Acupuncture," *Prev Med* 26, no. 1 (1997): 25-8.

[5] B. B. Abuaisha, J. B. Costanzi, and A. J. Boulton, "Acupuncture for the Treatment of Chronic Painful Peripheral Diabetic Neuropathy: A Long-Term Study," *Diabetes Res Clin Pr* 39, no. 2 (1998): 115-21.

[6] J. David et al., "Chronic Neck Pain: A Comparison of Acupuncture Treatment and Physiotherapy," *Brit J Rheumatol* 37, no. 10 (1998): 1118-22.

[7] R. Jensen et al., "Acupuncture Treatment of Patellofemoral Pain Syndrome," *J Altern Complem Med* 5, no. 6 (1999): 521-7.

[8] R. Mazzoni et al., "Failure of Acupuncture in the Treatment of Obesity: A Pilot Study," *Eating Weight Disorders* 4, no. 4 (1999): 198-202.

[9] J. Park, A. R. White, and E. Ernst, "Efficacy of Acupuncture as a Treatment for Tinnitus: A Systematic Review," *Arch Otolaryngol* 126, no. 4 (2000): 489-92.

[10] H. Honjo et al., "Acupuncture on Clinical Symptoms and Urodynamic Measurements in Spinal-Cord-Injured Patients with Detrusor Hyperreflexia," *Urol Int* 65, no. 4 (2000): 190-5.

[11] J. Roschke et al., "The Benefit from Whole Body Acupuncture in Major Depression," *J Affect Disorders* 57, nos. 1-3 (2000): 73-81.

[12] A. R. White et al., "Acupuncture for Episodic Tension-Type Headache: A Multicentre Randomized Controlled Trial," *Cephalalgia* 20, no. 7 (2000): 632-7.

[13] M. Karst et al., "Pressure Pain Threshold and Needle Acupuncture in Chronic Tension-Type Headache: A Double-Blind Placebo-Controlled Study," *Pain* 88, no. 2 (2000): 199-203.

[14] A. Margolin et al., "Acupuncture for the Treatment of Cocaine Addiction: A Randomized Controlled Trial," *J Amer Med Assoc* 287, no. 1 (2002): 55-63.

[15] A. R. White, H. Rampes, and E. Ernst, "Acupuncture for Smoking Cessation," *Cochrane Database of Systematic Reviews*, no. 2 (2000): CD000009.

TABLE B-3   REFLEXOLOGY—CLINICAL TRIAL

Year	Author	No.	Clinical Problem	Study Design/Comments	Help?
2000	White,[1] England	18	Diagnostic only	Tested ability of 2 experienced reflexologists to accurately diagnose 18 adults with ≥1 of 6 problems (neck pain, back pain, osteoarthritis of the knee, migraine, diabetes and sinusitis)	No
				All 6 conditions considered easily diagnosed per a reflexologist	
				2 reflexologists blinded to patients' diagnoses examined feet of each patient and rated the probability of which 6 conditions were present	

[1] A. R. White et al., "A Blinded Investigation into the Accuracy of Reflexology Charts," *Complement Ther Med* 8, no. 3 (2000): 166-72.

Table B-4   REFLEXOLOGY—CLINICAL TRIALS

Year	Author	No.	Clinical Problem	Study Design/Comments	Help?
1993	Oleson,[1] USA	35	Premenstrual symptoms	Study involved ear, hand and foot reflexology Controlled trial; placebo group received sham reflexology Both received 30 min. therapy/wk. for 8 wks. Both groups experienced relaxation Symptom diaries were recorded each day for 2 mos. prior to, during and after treatment (total 6 mos.)	Yes*
1997	Kesselring,[2] Germany	130	Voiding, pain, sleep, bowel movements and sense of well-being after abdominal surgery	*Majority of article was not translated into English, only the abstract (summary)* Controlled trial 3 groups: (1) foot reflexology (2) foot/leg massage (3) conversation Foot reflexology improved voiding but resulted in worse sleep Foot massage improved sense of well-being, sleep and pain Authors discourage foot reflexology for postoperative abdominal surgery patients	No
1999	Sudmeier,[3] Austria	32	Changes in blood flow to the kidneys while foot reflexology is being given to the kidney zone	*Majority of article was not translated into English, only the abstract (summary)* Controlled study with placebo group being treated in other foot zones Blood flow was measured using Doppler sonography, which measured velocity of blood flow and calculated the resistance Blood flow improved with reflexology (this was not a trial of the effect on disease)	N/A
2000	Stephenson,[4] USA	23	Anxiety and pain in patients with breast or lung cancer	Each patient given one real reflexology treatment and one sham treatment 30 min. each treatment	Yes**

CONTINUED ON NEXT PAGE

TABLE B-4 CONTINUED

Year	Author	No.	Clinical Problem	Study Design/Comments	Help?
2001	Brygge,[5] Denmark	40	Asthma	10 wks. of active or sham (placebo) reflexology	No
				While patients' symptoms improved (i.e., they thought they were breathing better), their objective lung-function tests did not change	
				Patients' symptoms improved on both real and sham reflexology. Symptom diaries indicated that some patients believed they were improving because they properly guessed that they were receiving genuine reflexology treatment	
				Lung-function tests did not improve on reflexology	
2002	Tovey,[6] England	34	Irritable bowel syndrome symptoms of abdominal pain, constipation/diarrhea and abdominal distention	Single-blind trial	No
				Randomized to 2 groups	
				Reflexology group: 6 30-min. sessions	
				Placebo group: nonreflexology foot massage 6 30-min. sessions	
				6 patients lost at 3 mos. follow-up—4 from reflexology and 2 from placebo	

*83 subjects began study; 48 dropped out (33 dropped 2 mos. prior to treatment; 15 dropped during treatment—7 from reflexology and 8 from placebo)

**This study used patients as own controls (crossover)

Except for the small study noted above, such research has not been forthcoming, as is evident in this table.

[1] T. Oleson and W. Flocco, "Randomized Controlled Study of Premenstrual Symptoms Treated with Ear, Hand, and Foot Reflexology," *Obstet Gynecol* 82, no. 6 (1993): 906-11.

[2] A. Kesselring, "Foot Reflexology Massage: A Clinical Study" (in German), *Forsch Komplementarmed* 6, no. 1 (1999): 38-40.

[3] I. Sudmeier et al., "Changes of Renal Blood Flow During Organ-Associated Foot Reflexology Measured by Color Doppler Sonography" (in German), *Forsch Komplementarmed* 6, no. 3 (1999): 129-34.

[4] N. L. Stephenson, S. P. Weinrich, and A. S. Tavakoli, "The Effects of Foot Reflexology on Anxiety and Pain in Patients with Breast and Lung Cancer," *Oncology Nursing Forum* 27, no. 1 (2000): 67-72.

CONTINUED ON NEXT PAGE

TABLE B-4 CONTINUED

[5] T. Brygge et al., "Reflexology and Bronchial Asthma," *Resp Med* 95, no. 3 (2001): 173-9.

[6] P. Tovey, "A Single-Blind Trial of Reflexology for Irritable Bowel Syndrome," *Brit J Gen Prac* 52, no. 474 (2002): 19-23.

TABLE B-5 APPLIED KINESIOLOGY—CLINICAL TRIALS

Year	Author	No.	Clinical Problem	Study Design/Comments	Help?
1988	Kenney,[1] USA	11	Ability of 3 AK practitioners to assess nutritional status	11 subjects tested for nutritional status of vitamins A, C, zinc and thiamin by (1) 3 experienced AK practitioners; (2) a dynamometer; and (3) laboratory AK practitioners did not agree with one another, the machine or the laboratory Double-blind: subjects given nutrients then tested by AK to see if deficient nutrient resulted in increased muscle strength	No
1993	Haas,[2] USA	42	Leg-length test for subluxation	Subjects were volunteers, staff, faculty and students from chiropractic college Subjects examined for subluxation in neck/thoracic spine Given either real or sham adjustment, then measured leg-length discrepancy for change	No
1993	Haas,[3] USA	42	Vertebral challenge test for leg-length discrepancy	Subjects were volunteers, staff, faculty and students from chiropractic college Double-blind; crossover Standardized rotatory force applied to specific vertebrae followed by exam of leg lengths	No

CONTINUED ON NEXT PAGE

TABLE B-5 CONTINUED

Year	Author	No.	Clinical Problem	Study Design/Comments	Help?
1994	Haas,[4] USA	68	Piriformis muscle strength during vertebral challenge test	Subjects were volunteers, staff, faculty and students from chiropractic college Tested whether or not piriformis muscle strength changed when a standardized force was applied sideways against spinous processes of T3-12 Piriformis strength was unaffected by challenge	No
1997	Lawson,[5] USA	32, 53	AK practitioners' agreement on muscle strength	3 experienced AK practitioners tested 2 different muscles for strength; they agreed upon piriformis but not upon hamstring strength Test repeated with 53 subjects and 2 other muscles; they agreed upon pectoralis but not tensor fascia lata	Yes and No
1998	Schmitt,[6] Israel	17	AK practitioners' ability to assess for food allergy	17 subjects tested positive for food allergies with AK muscle testing while food held in their mouths; then their blood was tested for allergies to same foods 90% of foods testing positive with AK also tested positive with RAST, IgE and IgG testing	Yes*
2001	Pothmann,[7] Germany	315	AK practitioners' ability to assess for food allergy	315 children with chronic disease (headache, abdominal pain, asthma, eczema) followed by AK x 2 yrs. AK tested against other AK practitioner (no agreement) and against laboratory allergy testing (RAST, IgG and lactose hydrogen breath tests; no agreement)	No

*Nonrandomized; nonblinded; noncontrolled

[1] J. J. Kenney, R. Clemens, and K. D. Forsythe, "Applied Kinesiology Unreliable for Assessing Nutrient Status," *J Am Diet Assoc* 88, no. 6 (1988): 698-704.

CONTINUED ON NEXT PAGE

TABLE B-5 CONTINUED

[2] M. Haas et al., "Responsiveness of Leg Alignment Changes Associated with Articular Pressure Testing to Spinal Manipulation: The Use of a Randomized Clinical Trial Design to Evaluate a Diagnostic Test with a Dichotomous Outcome [see comments]," *J Manip Physiol Ther* 16, no. 5 (1993): 306-11.

[3] M. Haas et al., "Reactivity of Leg Alignment to Articular Pressure Testing: Evaluation of a Diagnostic Test using a Randomized Crossover Clinical Trial Approach [see comments]," *J Manip Physiol Ther* 16, no. 4 (1993): 220-7.

[4] M. Haas et al., "Muscle Testing Response to Provocative Vertebral Challenge and Spinal Manipulation: A Randomized Controlled Trial of Construct Validity [see comments]," *J Manip Physiol Ther* 17, no. 3 (1994): 141-8.

[5] A. Lawson and L. Calderon, "Interexaminer Agreement for Applied Kinesiology Manual Muscle Testing," *Percept Mot Skills* 84, no. 2 (1997): 539-46.

[6] W. H. Schmitt, Jr., and G. Leisman, "Correlation of Applied Kinesiology Muscle Testing Findings with Serum Immunoglobulin Levels for Food Allergies," *Int J Neurosci* 96, nos. 3-4 (1998): 237-44.

[7] R. Pothmann et al., "Evaluation of Applied Kinesiology in Nutritional Intolerance of Childhood" (in German), *Forsch Komplementarmed Klass Naturheilkd* 8, no. 6 (2001): 336-44.

TABLE B-6   # CHELATION—CLINICAL TRIAL

Year	Author	No.	Clinical Problem	Study Design/Comments	Help?
2002	Knudtson,[1] USA	84	Coronary heart disease	Randomized; placebo-controlled; double-blind	No
				Participants had proven heart disease and an abnormal treadmill test	
				EDTA chelation or placebo treatment for 3 hrs., 2x/wk. x 15 wks., then 1x/mo. x 3	
				Both groups took vitamins by mouth	
				Treadmill test repeated at end of study period	

[1] M. L. Knudtson, "Chelation Therapy for Ischemic Heart Disease: A Randomized Controlled Trial," *J Amer Med Assoc* 287, no. 4 (2002): 481-6.

TABLE B-7   MAGNETIC THERAPY—CLINICAL TRIALS

Year	Author	No.	Clinical Problem	Study Design/Comments	Help?
1997	Vallbona,[1] USA	50	Postpolio pain	Randomized; double-blind; controlled Magnets or placebo magnets applied to affected areas for 45 min.	Yes
2000	Steyn,[2] USA	6	Blood flow in the feet of horses	Magnetic wrap applied to one leg x 48 hrs. Nonmagnetic wrap applied to opposite leg x 48 hrs. Blood flow of radioactive-tagged red blood cells measured before and after 48 hrs. of wrapping	No
2000	Collacott,[3] USA	20	Low back pain	Randomized; double-blind; controlled; crossover Magnets (or sham magnets) applied x 6 hr./d. every other d. for 1 wk. and then removed; then crossed over to other treatment for 1 wk.	No
2001	Alfano,[4] USA		Fibromyalgia	Randomized; controlled Tested benefit of magnetic sleep pads x 6 mos. 4 groups: 2 different magnetic sleep pads; 2 groups used sham sleep pads that looked/felt identical	No
2001	Mayrovitz,[5] USA	16	Blood flow to skin	Healthy female volunteers Magnets placed in 3 different positions on hand Sham magnet placed on opposite hand 36 min. duration for each Blood flow measured with Doppler techniques	No
2002	Carpenter,[6] USA	11	Hot flashes in breast cancer survivors	Randomized; double-blind; controlled; crossover Monitored hot flashes x 24 hrs., wore magnet or placebo x 3 d., off 10 d., crossed over	No

CONTINUED ON NEXT PAGE

TABLE B-7 CONTINUED

Year	Author	No.	Clinical Problem	Study Design/Comments	Help?
2002	Carter,[7] USA	30	Wrist pain in carpal tunnel syndrome	Randomized; double-blind; controlled Wrist wrap with a magnet x 45 min. v. same wrap with metal piece x 45 min.	No*
2002	Chaloupka,[8] USA	35	Hand muscle strength	Double-blind Grip strength tested (1) at baseline, (2) with placebo magnet, and (3) with genuine flexible magnet	No
2002	Segal,[9] USA/ Japan	64	Chronic knee pain in rheumatoid arthritis	Randomized; double-blind; controlled MagnaBloc v. control pad attached to knee for 1 wk.	No**

*Both improved

**Pain reduced in both groups (but not significantly more in MagnaBloc group)

[1] C. Vallbona, C. F. Hazlewood, and G. Jurida, "Response of Pain to Static Magnetic Fields in Postpolio Patients: A Double-Blind Pilot Study," *Arch Phys Med Rehabil* 78, no. 11 (1997): 1200-3.

[2] P. F. Steyn et al., "Effect of a Static Magnetic Field on Blood Flow to the Metacarpus in Horses," *J Am Vet Med Assoc* 217, no. 6 (2000): 874-7.

[3] E. A. Collacott, "Bipolar Permanent Magnets for the Treatment of Chronic Low Back Pain: A Pilot Study," *J Amer Med Assoc* 283, no. 10 (2000): 1322-5.

[4] A. P. Alfano et al., "Static Magnetic Fields for Treatment of Fibromyalgia: A Randomized Controlled Trial," *J Altern Complement Med* 7, no. 1 (2001): 53-64.

[5] H. N. Mayrovitz et al., "Effects of Permanent Magnets on Resting Skin Blood Perfusion in Healthy Persons Assessed by Laser Doppler Flowmetry and Imaging," *Bioelectromagnetics* 22, no. 7 (2001): 494-502.

[6] J. S. Carpenter et al., "A Pilot Study of Magnetic Therapy for Hot Flashes After Breast Cancer," *Cancer Nurse* 25, no. 2 (2002): 104-9.

[7] R. Carter, C. B. Aspy, and J. Mold, "The Effectiveness of Magnet Therapy for Treatment of Wrist Pain Attributed to Carpal Tunnel Syndrome," *J Fam Pract* 51, no. 1 (2002): 38-40.

[8] E. C. Chaloupka, J. Kang, and M. A. Mastrangelo, "The Effect of Flexible Magnets on Hand Muscle Strength: A Randomized, Double-Blind Study," *J Strength Cond Res* 16, no. 1 (2002): 33-7.

[9] N. A. Segal et al., "Two Configurations of Static Magnetic Fields for Treating Rheumatoid Arthritis of the Knee: A Double-Blind Clinical Trial," *Arch Phys Med Rehabil* 82, no. 10 (2001): 1453-60.

TABLE B-8   TOUCH THERAPY—CLINICAL TRIALS

Year	Author	No.	Clinical Problem	Study Design/Comments	Help?
1998	Rosa,[1] USA	15	TT Practitioners	See above Tested ability of TT practitioners to detect energy field near one of their hands	No
1998	Gordon,[2] USA	25	Osteoarthritis of the knee	Randomized; controlled; single-blind TT 1x/wk. x 6 wks. Placebo group received mock TT	Yes and No*
1998	Giasson,[3] USA	20	Sense of well-being in terminal cancer	Randomized; controlled TT given for 15 min. x 3 Control group allowed to rest x 3 Measured pain, nausea, depression, anxiety, etc.	Yes
1998	Turner,[4] USA	20	Low back pain	Randomized; double-blind; controlled; crossover Magnets (or sham magnets) applied x 6 hr./d. every other d. for 1 wk. and then removed; then crossed over to other treatment for 1 wk.	No
2001	Blankfield,[5] USA	21	Carpal tunnel syndrome	Randomized; single-blind TT 1x/wk. x 6 wks. v. sham TT Measured pain, relaxation and median nerve conduction	No

*Some measures of pain seemed to improve while others did not, nor did disability

[1] L. Rosa et al., "A Close Look at Therapeutic Touch," *J Amer Med Assoc* 279, no. 13 (1998): 1005-10.

[2] A. Gordon et al., "The Effects of Therapeutic Touch on Patients with Osteoarthritis of the Knee," *J Fam Pract* 47, no. 4 (1998): 271-7.

[3] M. Giasson and L. Bouchard, "Effect of Therapeutic Touch on the Well-Being of Persons with Terminal Cancer," *J Holist Nurs* 16, no. 3 (1998): 383-98.

[4] J. G. Turner et al., "The Effect of Therapeutic Touch on Pain and Anxiety in Burn Patients," *J Adv Nurs* 28, no. 1 (1998): 10-20.

[5] R. P. Blankfield et al., "Therapeutic Touch in the Treatment of Carpal Tunnel Syndrome," *J Am Board Fam Pract* 14, no. 5 (2001): 335-42.

ENDNOTES

Introduction
1. *Reader's Digest* (May 2002), p. 46.
2. *Arizona Republic* (May 2002), n.p.
3. Julie Appleby, *USA Today* (May 16, 2001), n.p.
4. J. Lazarou, B. H. Pomeranz and P. N. Corey, "Incidence of Adverse Drug Reactions in Hospitalized Patients: A Meta-Analysis of Prospective Studies," *Journal of the American Medical Association*, vol. 279, no. 15 (1998), pp. 1200-1205.
5. Thomas J. Moore, *Prescription for Disaster* (New York: Simon and Schuster, 1998), p. 115.
6. D. A. Kessler, "Introducing MedWatch," *Journal of the American Medical Association*, vol. 269 (1993), pp. 2765-2768.

Chapter One
1. *World Book Encyclopedia*, s.v. "Galileo."
2. Brian Inglis, *A History of Medicine* (Cleveland, OH: The World Publishing Company, 1965), p. 18.
3. Ibid., p. 21.
4. "The Soul of the Physician" (Journey into Wholeness conference brochure, Balsam Grove, NC, December 6-9, 2001).

Chapter Three
1. Brian Inglis, *A History of Medicine* (Cleveland, OH: The World Publishing Company, 1965), pp. 56-57.
2. Ibid., p. 54.
3. Ibid., p. 59.
4. For a further discussion on leprosy, see Dr. Paul Brand and Philip Yancey, *The Gift of Pain* (Zondervan, 1997). Dr. Paul Brand is a Christian missionary physician.

Chapter Four
1. Michael D. Jacobson, *The Word on Health* (Chicago, IL: Moody Press, 2000), pp. 21-33.

Chapter Five

1. Martin Seligman, *Learned Optimism* (New York: Pocket Books, 1990), pp. 65-66.
2. See Neil's book on anxiety disorders, which he coauthored with Rich Miller entitled *Freedom from Fear* (Eugene, OR: Harvest House, 1999).

   See also *Anger Kills* by Redford and Virginia Williams (New York: Harper Perennial, 1993). This is a secular book, but it reveals how our temperaments and anger can actually cause major illnesses and even death.
3. S. I. McMillen, M.D., *None of These Diseases* (Minneapolis, MN: Successful Living, Inc., 1963), p. 69.
4. Dr. Edmund J. Bourne, *The Anxiety and Phobia Workbook* (Oakland, CA: New Harbinger Publications, Inc., 1995), n.p.
5. Dr. Edmund J. Bourne, *Healing Fear* (Oakland, CA: New Harbinger Publications, Inc., 1998), p. 2.
6. Ibid., p. 3.
7. Ibid., p. 5.

Chapter Six

1. *Dorland's Illustrated Medical Dictionary,* 26th ed., s.v. "science."
2. Ibid.
3. *World Book Encyclopedia,* s.v. "scientific method."
4. Peter Marshall and David Manuel, *The Light and the Glory* (Grand Rapids, MI: Fleming H. Revell, 1992), p. 14.
5. J. Krop et al., "A Double-Blind, Randomized, Controlled Investigation of Electrodermal Testing in the Diagnosis of Allergies," *Jouranl of Alternative and Complementary Medicine,* vol. 3, no. 3 (1997), pp. 241-248.
6. G. T. Lewith et al., "Is Electrodermal Testing As Effective As Skin Prick Tests for Diagnosing Allergies? A Double Blind, Randomized Block Design Study," *British Medical Journal,* vol. 322, no. 7279 (2001), pp. 131-134.
7. James P. Carter, "If EDTA Chelation Therapy Is So Good, Why Is It Not More Widely Accepted?" *Journal of Advancement in Medicine,* vol. 2 $^1/_2$ (1989), pp. 213-226.

Chapter Seven

1. Hari M. Sharma, "Maharishi Ayurveda," in *Fundamentals of Complementary and Alternative Medicine,* ed. Marc S. Micozzi (New York: Churchill Livingstone, 1996), pp. 243-57.
2. Ted J. Kaptchuk, "Historical Context of the Concept of Vitalism," in *Fundamentals of Complementary and Alternative Medicine,* ed. Marc S. Micozzi (New York: Churchill Livingstone, 1995), pp. 35-48.
3. Brian Inglis, *A History of Medicine* (Cleveland, OH: The World Publishing Company, 1965), pp. 121-124.
4. Paul C. Reisser, Dale Mabe and Robert Velarde, *Examining Alternative Medicine: An Inside Look at the Benefits and Risks* (Downers Grove, IL: InterVarsity Press, 2001), pp. 109-110.
5. Kaptchuk, "Historical Context of the Concept of Vitalism," in *Fundamentals of Complementary and Alternative Medicine,* pp. 35-48.

6. Ibid.

7. Victoria E. Slater, "Healing Touch," in *Fundamentals of Complementary and Alternative Medicine,* ed. Marc S. Micozzi (New York: Churchill Livingstone, 1995), pp. 121-36.

8. *Wycliffe Bible Commentary* (Willow Grove, PA: Woodlawn Electronic Publishing, ©Tri Star Publishing, 1988), n.p.

Chapter Eight

1. How blessed we are to have modern-day examples like Doctors David Stevens and Paul Brand, who, like Elisha, forsook worldly riches in order that the grace of God might be freely given to those in need. Dr. Stevens served in Africa as a missionary doctor and is now the executive director of the Christian Medical and Dental Society. (We highly recommend his book *Jesus, M.D.,* Zondervan, 2001.) Dr. Paul Brand served for years in India as a missionary doctor and coauthored several outstanding books with Philip Yancey, including *The Gift of Pain, Fearfully and Wonderfully Made* and *In His Image,* all published by Zondervan. And there are many other godly doctors who serve the needs of people everywhere, with Christian motives and compassion.

2. Doctors and nurses are fallible. It is estimated that at least 100,000 people die every year of medical malpractice. Our health and well-being is a huge responsibility they carry. But it is still our responsibility to discern God's direction for our treatments. Once determined, we should pray for our health-care providers, our doctors and people undergoing anesthesia. Patients under anesthesia are voluntarily surrendering the use of their minds. In such a passive state, they are spiritually vulnerable. We should ask God for spiritual protection and that He would enable the surgical team to operate with wisdom and skill.

3. Kevin V. Ergil, "China's Traditional Medicine," in *Fundamentals of Complementary and Alternative Medicine,* ed. Marc S. Micozzi (New York: Churchill Livingstone, 1995), p. 212.

Chapter Nine

1. Maharishi Mahesh Yogi et al., *Fundamentals of Maharishi Ayur-Ved: A Personalized Guide for Diet and Seasonal and Daily Routines* (Colorado Springs, CO: Maharishi Ayur-Ved Products International, 1995), p. 1.

2. Hari M. Sharma, "Maharishi Ayurveda," in *Fundamentals of Complementary and Alternative Medicine,* ed. Marc S. Micozzi (New York: Churchill Livingstone, 1996), p. 243.

3. *Grolier's Encyclopedia,* s.v. "Vedas."

4. William Collinge, *The American Holistic Health Association Complete Guide to Alternative Medicine* (New York: Warner Books, 1987), p. 55.

5. Kenneth G. Zysk, "Ayurveda Medicine," in *Fundamentals of Complementary and Alternative Medicine,* ed. Marc S. Micozzi (New York: Churchill Livingstone, 1996), p. 233.

6. Sharma, "Maharishi Ayurveda," in *Fundamentals of Complementary and Alternative Medicine,* pp. 243-247.

7. Collinge, *The American Holistic Health Association Complete Guide to Alternative Medicine,* p. 57.

8. Dónal O'Mathúna and Walt Larimore, *Alternative Medicine: The Christian Handbook* (Grand Rapids, MI: Zondervan, 2001), p. 155.

9. Sharma, "Maharishi Ayurveda," in *Fundamentals of Complementary and Alternative Medicine*, p. 245.

10. Ibid.

11. *Grolier's Encyclopedia*, s.v. "pure intelligence."

12. *Grolier's Encyclopedia*, s.v. "hinduism."

13. Collinge, *The American Holistic Health Association Complete Guide to Alternative Medicine*, p. 58.

14. Zysk, "Ayurveda Medicine," in *Fundamentals of Complementary and Alternative Medicine*, pp. 233-234.

15. Sharma, "Maharishi Ayurveda," in *Fundamentals of Complementary and Alternative Medicine*, p. 248.

16. Collinge, *The American Holistic Health Association Complete Guide to Alternative Medicine*, p. 62.

17. Sharma, "Maharishi Ayurveda," in *Fundamentals of Complementary and Alternative Medicine*, pp. 247-250.

18. Collinge, *The American Holistic Health Association Complete Guide to Alternative Medicine*, p. 62.

19. Zysk, "Ayurveda Medicine," in *Fundamentals of Complementary and Alternative Medicine*, pp. 237-240.

20. O'Mathuna and Larimore, *Alternative Medicine: The Christian Handbook*, p. 156.

21. Yogi, *Fundamentals of Maharishi Ayur-Ved: A Personalized Guide for Diet and Seasonal and Daily Routines*, p. 2.

22. Sharma, "Maharishi Ayurveda," in *Fundamentals of Complementary and Alternative Medicine*, p. 246.

23. *Grolier's Encyclopedia*, s.v. "siddhis."

24. Collinge, *The American Holistic Health Association Complete Guide to Alternative Medicine*, p. 75.

25. Isadore Rosenfeld, M.D., *Dr. Rosenfeld's Guide to Alternative Medicine* (New York: Fawcett Books), p. 65.

26. Sanjay Kumar, "Indian Herbal Remedies Come Under Attack," *Lancet*, vol. 351 (April 1998), p. 1190.

27. O'Mathuna and Larimore, *Alternative Medicine: The Christian Handbook*, pp. 286-287.

28. M. S. Garfinkel et al., "Yoga-Based Intervention for Carpal Tunnel Syndrome: A Randomized Trial," *Journal of the American Medical Association*, vol. 280 (1998), pp. 1601-1603.

29. O'Mathuna and Larimore, *Alternative Medicine: The Christian Handbook*, pp. 247-249.

30. L. Bernardi et al., "Effect of Rosary Prayer and Yoga Mantras on Autonomic Cardiovascular Rhythms: Comparative Study," *British Medical Journal*, vol. 323, no. 7327 (2001), pp. 1446-1449.

31. Sharma, "Maharishi Ayurveda," in *Fundamentals of Complementary and Alternative Medicine*, pp. 246-247.

32. O'Mathuna and Larimore, *Alternative Medicine: The Christian Handbook*, p. 247.

33. *Grolier's Encyclopedia*, s.v. "yoga."

34. "How to Begin and Maintain Meditation" (Institute in Basic Life Principles seminar booklet, Oakbridge, IL, 1987).

35. Sharma, "Maharishi Ayurveda," in *Fundamentals of Complementary and Alternative Medicine*, p. 245.

Chapter Ten

1. Richard Haehl, *Samuel Hahnemann: His Life and Work,* trans. Marie L. Wheeler and W. H. R. Grundy, 2 vols. (New Delhi, India: B. Jain Publishers Pvt. Ltd., 1992), p. 67.
2. *Dorland's Illustrated Medical Dictionary,* 26th ed., s.v. "allopathy."
3. *World Book Encyclopedia,* s.v. "Hippocrates."
4. Inglis, *A History of Medicine,* p. 97.
5. Martin Gumpert, *Hahnemann: The Adventurous Career of a Medical Rebel* (New York: L. B. Fischer, 1945), pp. 115-116.
6. Martin Kaufman, *Homeopathy in America: The Rise and Fall of a Medical Heresy* (Baltimore, MD: Johns Hopkins Press, 1971), p. 7.
7. George Wald, *Frontiers of Modern Biology on Theories of Origin of Life* (New York: Houghton Mifflin, 1972), p. 187.
8. *Dorland's Illustrated Medical Dictionary,* 26th ed., s.v. "allopathy."
9. J. Lazarou, B. H. Pomeranz and P. N. Corey, "Incidence of Adverse Drug Reactions in Hospitalized Patients: A Meta-Analysis of Prospective Studies," *Journal of the American Medical Association,* vol. 279, no. 15 (1998), pp. 1200-1205.

Chapter Eleven

1. Andrew T. Still, *Philosophy of Osteopathy* (Kirksville, MO: A. T. Still, 1899), p. 15.
2. *Dorland's Illustrated Medical Dictionary,* 26th ed., s.v. "osteopathy."
3. Still, *Philosophy of Osteopathy,* p. iii.
4. Still, *Philosophy of Osteopathy,* p. ii.
5. Still, *Philosophy of Osteopathy,* pp. 27-28.
6. G. B. Anderson et al., "A Comparison of Osteopathic Spinal Manipulation with Standard Care for Patients with Low Back Pain," *New England Journal of Medicine,* vol. 341, no. 19 (1999), pp. 1426-1431.

    R. S. MacDonald and C. M. Bell, "An Open Controlled Assessment of Osteopathic Manipulation in Nonspecific Low-Back Pain," *Spine,* vol. 15, no. 5 (1990), pp. 364-370.

    G. Bronfort et al., "Efficacy of Spinal Manipulation for Chronic Headache: A Systematic Review," *Journal of Manipulative and Physiological Therapeutics,* vol. 24, no. 7 (2001), pp. 457-466.

    A. K. Burton, K. M. Tillotson and J. Cleary, "Single-Blind Randomised Controlled Trial of Chemonucleolysis and Manipulation in the Treatment of Symptomatic Lumbar Disc Herniation," *European Spine Journal,* vol. 9, no. 3 (2000), pp. 202-207.
7. M. A. Hondras, K. Linde and A. P. Jones, "Manual Therapy for Asthma," *Cochrane Database of Systematic Reviews,* no. 1 (2001), p. CD001002.
8. R. Jarski et al., "The Effectiveness of Osteopathic Manipulative Treatment as Complementary Therapy Following Surgery: A Prospective, Match-Controlled Outcome Study," *Alternative Therapies in Health and Medicine,* vol. 6, no. 5 (2000), pp. 77-81.
9. D. R. Noll et al., "Benefits of Osteopathic Manipulative Treatment for Hospitalized Elderly Patients with Pneumonia," *Journal of the American Osteopathic Association,* vol. 100, no. 12 (2000), pp. 776-782.
10. C. Green et al., "A Systematic Review of Craniosacral Therapy: Biological Plausibility, Assessment Reliability and Clinical Effectiveness," *Complementary Therapies in Medicine,* vol. 7, no. 4 (1999), pp. 201-207.

Kenneth R. Pelletier, *The Best Alternative Medicine* (New York: Simon and Schuster, 2001), n.p.

11. W. P. Hanten et al., "Craniosacral Rhythm: Reliability and Relationships with Cardiac and Respiratory Rates," *Journal of Orthopaedic and Sports Physical Therapy*, vol. 27, no. 3 (1998), pp. 213-218.

R. W. Moran and P. Gibbons, "Intraexaminer and Interexaminer Reliability for Palpation of the Cranial Rhythmic Impulse at the Head and Sacrum," *Journal of Manipulative and Physiological Therapeutics*, vol. 24, no. 3 (2001), pp. 183-190.

J. S. Rogers et al., "Simultaneous Palpation of the Craniosacral Rate at the Head and Feet: Intrarater and Interrater Reliability and Rate Comparisons," *Physical Therapy*, vol. 78, no. 11 (1998), pp. 1175-1185.

12. J. M. McPartland and E. A. Mein, "Entrainment and the Cranial Rhythmic Impulse," *Alternative Therapies in Health and Medicine*, vol. 3, no. 1 (1997), pp. 40-45.

Chapter Twelve

1. Isadore Rosenfeld, *Dr. Rosenfeld's Guide to Alternative Medicine* (New York: Random House, 1996), p. 106.
2. D. D. Palmer, *The Science, Art and Philosophy of Chiropractic*, 5th ed., *Chiropractor's Adjuster* (Davenport, IA: The Palmer School of Chiropractic Publishers, 1920), p. 17.
3. Palmer, *The Science, Art and Philosophy of Chiropractic*, p. 20.
4. William Collinge, *The American Holistic Health Association Complete Guide to Alternative Medicine* (New York: Warner Books, 1987), p. 234.
5. Martin Kauf, *Homeopathy in America: The Rise and Fall of a Medical Heresy* (Baltimore, MD: Johns Hopkins Press, 1971), p. 90.
6. Daniel Redwood, "Chiropractic," in *Fundamentals of Complementary and Alternative Medicine*, ed. Marc S. Micozzi (New York: Churchill Livingstone, 1995), p. 93.
7. Redwood, "Chiropractic," in *Fundamentals of Complementary and Alternative Medicine*, p. 95.
8. Palmer, *The Science, Art and Philosophy of Chiropractic*, p. 17.
9. Ibid.
10. *Dorland's Illustrated Medical Dictionary*, 26th ed., s.v. "chiropractic."
11. Palmer, *The Science, Art and Philosophy of Chiropractic*, p. 19.
12. Redwood, "Chiropractic," in *Fundamentals of Complementary and Alternative Medicine*, p. 92.
13. Ibid., pp. 92, 97.
14. I. M. Korr, "Sustained Sympathicotonia as a Factor in Disease," in *The Neurobiologic Mechanisms in Manipulative Therapy* (New York: Penguin Press, 1977), pp. 229-258.
15. Redwood, "Chiropractic," in *Fundamentals of Complementary and Alternative Medicine*, p. 96.
16. Kenneth R. Pelletier, *The Best Alternative Medicine* (New York: Simon and Schuster, 2001), pp. 222-223.
17. Redwood, "Chiropractic," in *Fundamentals of Complementary and Alternative Medicine*, p. 104.
18. Pelletier, *The Best Alternative Medicine*, p. 226.
19. Rosenfeld, *Dr. Rosenfeld's Guide to Alternative Medicine*, p. 109.
20. Collinge, *The American Holistic Health Association Complete Guide to Alternative Medicine*, p. 96.

21. Joseph E. Pizzorno, Jr., "Naturopathic Medicine," in *Fundamentals of Complementary and Alternative Medicine,* ed. Marc S. Micozzi (New York: Churchill Livingstone, 1995), pp. 163-181.

22. Collinge, *The American Holistic Health Association Complete Guide to Alternative Medicine,* pp. 109-112.

23. Rosenfeld, *Dr. Rosenfeld's Guide to Alternative Medicine,* p. 221.

24. Josef M. Issels, "Immunotherapy in Cancer," *Explore,* vol. 7, no. 6 (1997), n.p.

25. Pizzorno, "Naturopathic Medicine," in *Fundamentals of Complementary and Alternative Medicine,* p. 178.

26. Rosenfeld, *Dr. Rosenfeld's Guide to Alternative Medicine,* p. 221.

27. R. Kleef et al., "Fever, Cancer Incidence and Spontaneous Remissions," *Neuroimmunomodulation,* vol. 9, no. 2 (2001), pp. 55-64.

28. S. Ohno et al., "Hyperthermia for Rectal Cancer," *Surgery,* vol. 131, no. 1 (2002), pp. 121-127.

29. T. Kerner et al., "Whole Body Hyperthermia: A Secure Procedure for Patients with Various Malignancies?" *Intensive Care Medicine,* vol. 25, no. 9 (1999), pp. 959-965.

30. Rosenfeld, *Dr. Rosenfeld's Guide to Alternative Medicine,* pp. 221-222.

31. Elias Ilyia, "Melatonin Assessment" (paper presented at the Gastrointestinal Diagnosis and Melatonin Assessment, Oak Brook, IL, June 14-15, 1997).

32. P. N. Karnauchow, "Melanoma and Sun Exposure," *Lancet,* vol. 346 (1995), p. 915.

33. Gregory Maltz, "Sunlight May Protect Against Cancers, Melanoma," *Family Practice News* (1996), p. 21.

34. Rex Russell, "A Biblical Perspective on Diet" (live presentation at the Coronary Atheroma Regression Evaluation (CARE), Christ Hospital, Cincinnati, OH, January 15, 1997).

35. Mark A. Newman, "Tans Can Protect Against Melanoma," *Skin and Allergy News* (1996), p. 10.

36. K. G. Thampy, "Hypercholesterolaemia of Prolonged Fasting and Cholesterol Lowering of Re-Feeding in Lean Human Subjects," *Scandinavian Journal of Clinical and Laboratory Investigation,* vol. 55, no. 4 (1995), pp. 351-357.

37. E. Ernst, "Colonic Irrigation and the Theory of Autointoxication: A Triumph of Ignorance over Science," *Journal of Clinical Gastroenterology,* vol. 24, no. 4 (1997), pp. 196-198.

Chapter Thirteen

1. *Dorland's Illustrated Medical Dictionary,* 26th ed., s.v. "homeopathy."

2. Francisco Xavier Eizayaga, *Treatise on Homeopathic Medicine,* 3rd ed. (Buenos Aires: Ediciones Marecel, 1991), p. 29.

3. Ibid.

4. Richard Haehl, *Samuel Hahnemann: His Life and Work,* trans. Marie L. Wheeler and W. H. R. Grundy, 2 vols. (New Delhi, India: B. Jain Publishers Pvt. Ltd., 1992), pp. 36-37.

5. Ibid.

6. Eizayaga, *Treatise on Homeopathic Medicine,* p. 49.

7. Haehl, *Samuel Hahnemann: His Life and Work,* pp. 36-38, 99-104.

8. Eizayaga, *Treatise on Homeopathic Medicine,* p. 29.
      Haehl, *Samuel Hahnemann: His Life and Work,* pp. 1-9, 26-40.

9. Haehl, *Samuel Hahnemann: His Life and Work,* pp. 390-391.

10. Ibid., p. 25.
11. Ibid., pp. 95-99.
12. Ibid.
13. Ibid., p. 67.
14. Ibid., pp. 136-152.
15. Rima Handley, *A Homeopathic Love Story: The Story of Samuel and Mélanie Hahnemann* (Berkeley, CA: North Atlantic Books, 1990), pp. 153-156.
    Haehl, *Samuel Hahnemann: His Life and Work*, pp. 242-245, 355-361.
16. Haehl, *Samuel Hahnemann: His Life and Work*, pp. 251-254, 388-389.
17. Ibid., p. 387.
18. Handley, *A Homeopathic Love Story: The Story of Samuel and Mélanie Hahnemann*, p. 9.
19. Haehl, *Samuel Hahnemann: His Life and Work*, pp. 251-252.
20. Samuel Pfeifer, M.D., *Healing at Any Price* (Milton Keynes, England: Word Limited, 1988), n.p.
21. Eizayaga, *Treatise on Homeopathic Medicine*, pp. 45-46.
22. Haehl, *Samuel Hahnemann: His Life and Work*, p. 6.
23. Ibid., p. 81.
24. Eizayaga, *Treatise on Homeopathic Medicine*, pp. 18-19.
    Haehl, *Samuel Hahnemann: His Life and Work*, p. 67.
25. Jennifer Jacobs and Richard Moskowitz, "Homeopathy," in *Fundamentals of Complementary and Alternative Medicine*, ed. Marc S. Miccozi (New York: Churchill Livingstone, 1995), pp. 67-78.
26. John Ankerberg and John Weldon, *Can You Trust Your Doctor?* (Brentwood, TN: Wolgemuth and Hyatt, 1991), pp. 19, 273.
    Haehl, *Samuel Hahnemann: His Life and Work*, p. 272.
27. Martin Gumpert, *Hahnemann: The Adventurous Career of a Medical Rebel* (New York: L. B. Fischer, 1945), p. 89.
28. Haehl, *Samuel Hahnemann: His Life and Work*, p. 330.
29. Ibid., pp. 266-267.
30. Martin Kaufman, *Homeopathy in America: The Rise and Fall of a Medical Heresy* (Baltimore, MD: Johns Hopkins Press, 1971), pp. 110, 122-123.
31. Haehl, *Samuel Hahnemann: His Life and Work*, p. 436.
32. Ankerberg and Weldon, *Can You Trust Your Doctor?* pp. 36-40.
33. Adelaide Suits, *Brass Tacks: Oral Biography of a Twentieth Century Physician* (Ann Arbor, MI: Halyburton Press, 1985), p. 21.
    Haehl, *Samuel Hahnemann: His Life and Work*, pp. 310-345.
34. H. Walach, "Does a Highly Diluted Homeopathic Drug Act as a Placebo in Healthy Volunteers? Experimental Study of Belladonna 30c in Double-Blind Crossover Design—a Pilot Study," *Journal of Psychosomatic Research*, vol. 37, no. 8 (1993), pp. 851-860.
35. M. A. Taylor et al., "Randomized Controlled Trial of Homeopathy Versus Placebo in Perennial Allergic Rhinitis with Overview of Four Trial Series," *British Medical Journal*, vol. 321, no. 7259 (2000), pp. 471-476.
36. Pfeifer, *Healing at Any Price*, n.p.
37. Jacobs and Moskowitz, "Homeopathy," in *Fundamentals of Complementary and Alternative Medicine*, pp. 67-78.
38. Peter Fisher, "Homeopathy, a Scientific Update" (paper presented at the World Med '96, Washington, DC, May 25, 1996).

39. Jos Kleijnen et al., "Clinical Trials of Homeopathy," *British Medical Journal* (1991), pp. 302-323.
40. Kathryn Senior, "Homeopathy: Science or Scam?" *Molecular Medicine Today* (1995), pp. 266-269.
41. Eizayaga, *Treatise on Homeopathic Medicine,* p. 29.
42. Gumpert, *Hahnemann: The Adventurous Career of a Medical Rebel,* pp. 123-124.
43. Eizayaga, *Treatise on Homeopathic Medicine,* p. 31.
44. Haehl, *Samuel Hahnemann: His Life and Work,* pp. 159-166, 190-191.
45. Pfeifer, *Healing at Any Price,* n.p.
46. Samuel Hahnemann and Edward Hamlyn, *The Healing Art of Homeopathy* (New Canaan, CT: Keats Publishing, 1981), p. 15.
47. Haehl, *Samuel Hahnemann: His Life and Work,* p. 126.

Chapter Fourteen

1. Kevin V. Ergil, "China's Traditional Medicine," in *Fundamentals of Complementary and Alternative Medicine,* ed. Marc S. Micozzi (New York: Churchill Livingstone, 1995), pp. 185-223.
2. Ergil, "China's Traditional Medicine," in *Fundamentals of Complementary and Alternative Medicine,* p. 193.
3. *World Book Encyclopedia,* s.v. "Taoism."
4. Samuel Pfeifer, M.D., *Healing at Any Price* (Milton Keynes, England: Word Limited, 1988), n.p.
5. Ergil, "China's Traditional Medicine," in *Fundamentals of Complementary and Alternative Medicine,* p. 197.
6. Ibid., p. 199.
7. Ibid., p. 201.
8. Ibid., p. 205.
9. Ibid., p. 206.
10. Charles T. McGee, Kenneth Sancier and Effie Poy Yew Chow, "Qigong in Traditional Chinese Medicine," in *Fundamentals of Complementary and Alternative Medicine,* ed. Marc S. Micozzi (New York: Churchill Livingstone, 1995), pp. 225-230.
11. Roger Jahnke, "Qigong and Tai Chi: China's Self Healing Arts" (paper presented at the World Med '96, Washington, DC, May 24, 1996).
12. Ergil, "China's Traditional Medicine," in *Fundamentals of Complementary and Alternative Medicine,* p. 206.
13. M. T. Wu et al., "Central Nervous Pathway for Acupuncture Stimulation: Localization of Processing with Functional MR Imaging of the Brain—Preliminary Experience," *Radiology,* vol. 212, no. 1 (1999), pp. 133-141.
14. E. Haker, H. Egekvist and P. Bjerring, "Effect of Sensory Stimulation (Acupuncture) on Sympathetic and Parasympathetic Activities in Healthy Subjects," *Journal of the Autonomic Nervous System,* vol. 79, no. 1 (2000), pp. 52-59.
15. Ronald Melzack, "How Acupuncture Works: A Sophisticated Western Theory Takes the Mystery Out," *Psychology Today* (June 1973), p. 34.
16. Charles Owens, *An Endocrine Interpretation of Chapman's Reflexes,* 2nd ed. (Colorado Springs, CO: American Academy of Osteopathy, 1937), p. 2.
17. George S. Hackett, *Ligament and Tendon Relaxation Treated by Prolotherapy,* 3rd ed. (Springfield, IL: Charles C. Thomas, 1958), p. 27.

18. Ergil, "China's Traditional Medicine," in *Fundamentals of Complementary and Alternative Medicine*, p. 219.
19. Eva Haker, R.P.T., and Thomas Lundeberg, M.D., Ph.D., "Acupuncture Treatment in Epicondylalgia: A Comparative Study of Two Acupuncture Techniques," *Clinical Journal of Pain*, vol. 6, no. 3 (1990), pp. 221-226.
20. J. Kleijnen et al., "Acupuncture and Asthma: A Review of Controlled Trials," *Thorax*, vol. 46 (1991), pp. 799-802.
21. Dónal O'Mathúna and Walt Larimore, *Alternative Medicine: The Christian Handbook* (Grand Rapids, MI: Zondervan Publishing House, 2001), pp. 147-150.
22. Ergil, "China's Traditional Medicine," in *Fundamentals of Complementary and Alternative Medicine*, p. 219.
23. M. Girodo, K. A. Ekstrand and G. J. Metivier, "Deep Diaphragmatic Breathing: Rehabilitation Exercises for the Asthmatic Patient," *Archives of Physical Medicine and Rehabilitation*, vol. 73, no. 8 (1992), pp. 717-720.
24. Q. Yan and Y. Sun, "Quantitative Research for Improving Respiratory Muscle Contraction by Breathing Exercise," *Chinese Medical Journal*, vol. 109, no. 10 (1996), pp. 771-775.
25. McGee, "Qigong in Traditional Chinese Medicine," in *Fundamentals of Complementary and Alternative Medicine*, p. 228.
26. T. Hisamitsu et al., "Emission of Extremely Strong Magnetic Fields from the Head and Whole Body During Oriental Breathing Exercises," *Acupuncture and Electro-Therapeutics Research*, vol. 21, nos. 3-4 (1996), pp. 219-227.
27. J. Z. Zhang, J. Zhao and Q. N. He, "EEG Findings During Special Psychical State (Qi Gong State) by Means of Compressed Spectral Array and Topographic Mapping," *Computers in Biology and Medicine*, vol. 18, no. 6 (1988), pp. 455-463.
28. McGee, "Qigong in Traditional Chinese Medicine," in *Fundamentals of Complementary and Alternative Medicine*, p. 227.
29. Ibid., p. 228.
30. X. F. Lei et al., "The Antitumor Effects of Qigong-Emitted External Qi and Its Influence on the Immunologic Functions of Tumor-Bearing Mice," *Journal of Tongji Medical University*, vol. 11, no. 4 (1991), pp. 253-256.
31. Y. A. Lim et al., "Effects of Qigong on Cardiorespiratory Changes: A Preliminary Study," *American Journal of Chinese Medicine*, vol. 21, no. 1 (1993), pp. 1-6.
   H. Ryu et al., "Effect of Qigong Training on Proportions of T Lymphocyte Subsets in Human Peripheral Blood," *American Journal of Chinese Medicine*, vol. 23, no. 1 (1995), pp. 27-36.
   H. Ryu et al., "Delayed Cutaneous Hypersensitivity Reactions in Qigong (Chun Do Sun Bup) Trainees by Multitest Cell Mediated Immunity," *American Journal of Chinese Medicine*, vol. 23, no. 2 (1995), pp. 139-144.
32. McGee, "Qigong in Traditional Chinese Medicine," in *Fundamentals of Complementary and Alternative Medicine*, p. 227.
33. D. P. Wirth, J. R. Cram and R. J. Chang, "Multisite Electromyographic Analysis of Therapeutic Touch and Qigong Therapy," *Journal of Alternate and Complementary Medicine*, vol. 3, no. 2 (1997), pp. 109-118.
34. Mary Austin, *The Textbook of Acupuncture Therapy* (New York, NY: ASI Publishers, Inc., 1978), pp. 49-51.
35. McGee, "Qigong in Traditional Chinese Medicine," in *Fundamentals of Complementary and Alternative Medicine*, p. 229.

36. Y. Omura and S. L. Beckman, "Application of Intensified (+) Qi Gong Energy, (-) Electrical Field, (S) Magnetic Field, Electrical Pulses (1-2 Pulses/Sec.), Strong Shiatsu Massage or Acupuncture on the Accurate Organ Representation Areas of the Hands to Improve Circulation and Enhance Drug Uptake in Pathological Organs: Clinical Applications with Special Emphasis on the 'Chlamydia-(Lyme)-Uric Acid Syndrome' and 'Chlamydia-(Cytomegalovirus)-Uric Acid Syndrome,'" *Acupuncture and Electro-Therapeutics Research,* vol. 20, no. 1 (1995), pp. 21-72.

37. Ibid.

38. H. H. Shan et al., "Clinical Phenomenology of Mental Disorders Caused by Qigong Exercise," *Chinese Medical Journal,* vol. 102, no. 6 (1989), pp. 445-448.

39. S. H. Xu, "Psychophysiological Reactions Associated with Qigong Therapy," *Chinese Medical Journal,* vol. 107, no. 3 (1994), pp. 230-233.

40. Reisser et al., "Comparisons of Pain Relief Mechanisms Between Needling to the Muscle, Static Magnetic Field, External Qigong and Needling to the Acupuncture Point," *Acupuncture and Electro-Therapeutics Research,* vol. 21, no. 2 (1996), pp. 119-131.

41. Everett Ferguson, *Demonology of the Early Christian World* (New York: Edwin Mellen Press, 1985), pp. 116-117.

Chapter Fifteen

1. *Dorland's Illustrated Medical Dictionary,* 26th ed., s.v. "iridology."

2. Brian Inglis and Ruth West, *The Alternative Health Guide* (New York: Alfred A. Knopf, 1983), p. 279.

3. Samuel Pfeifer, M.D., *Healing at Any Price* (Milton Keynes, England: Word Limited, 1988), n.p.

4. John Ankerberg and John Weldon, *Can You Trust Your Doctor?* (Brentwood, TN: Wolgemuth and Hyatt, 1991), p. 342.

5. Brian Inglis, *A History of Medicine* (Cleveland, OH: The World Publishing Company, 1965), pp. 72-79.

6. Paul C. Reisser, Teri K. Reisser and John Weldon, *New Age Medicine: A Christian Perspective on Holistic Health* (Downers Grove, IL: InterVarsity Press, 1988), p. 144.

7. Ankerberg and Weldon, *Can You Trust Your Doctor?* p. 345.

8. Pfeifer, *Healing at Any Price,* n.p.

9. Ibid., pp. 89-90.

10. P. Knipschild, "Looking for Gall Bladder Disease in the Patient's Iris," *British Medical Journal,* vol. 297, no. 6663 (1988), pp. 1578-1581.

11. T. J. Buchanan et al., "An Investigation of the Relationship Between Anatomical Features in the Iris and Systemic Disease, with Reference to Iridology," *Complementary Therapies in Medicine,* vol. 4, no. 2 (1996), pp. 98-102.

12. Allie Simon, David M. Worthen and John A. Mitas, "An Evaluation of Iridology," *Journal of the American Medical Association,* vol. 242 (September 28, 1979), pp. 1385-1389.

13. Ankerberg and Weldon, *Can You Trust Your Doctor?* p. 342.

14. Simon, Worthen and Mita, "An Evaluation of Iridology," pp. 1385-1389.

15. Ankerberg and Weldon, *Can You Trust Your Doctor?* p. 354.

16. Kurt Koch, *The Devil's Alphabet* (Grand Rapids, MI: Kregel Publications, 1969), pp. 40-41.

17. *Dorland's Illustrated Medical Dictionary*, 26th ed., s.v. "reflexology."
18. Burton Goldberg Group, Alternative Medicine: The Definitive Guide (Fife, WA: Future Medicine Publishing, Inc., 1993), p. 108.
19. Michael D. Jacobson, "Traditional Chinese Medicine," *Simply Providential*, vol. 1, no. 4 (1998), p. 7.
20. Inglis and West, *The Alternative Health Guide*, pp. 112-113.
21. Ibid.
22. Charles Owens, *An Endocrine Interpretation of Chapman's Reflexes*, 2nd ed. (Colorado Springs, CO: American Academy of Osteopathy, 1937), pp. 26-27.
23. A. R. White et al., "A Blinded Investigation into the Accuracy of Reflexology Charts," *Complementary Therapies in Medicine*, vol. 8, no. 3 (2000), pp. 166-172.

Chapter Sixteen
1. Brian Inglis and Ruth West, *The Alternative Health Guide* (New York: Alfred A. Knopf, 1983), p. 116.
2. George J. Goodheart, "Chiropractic Applied Kinesiology" (paper presented at the Introduction to Complementary Alternative Medicine, Wayne State University School of Medicine, Detroit, MI, 1999).
3. R. H. Gin and B. N. Green, "George Goodheart, Jr., D.C., and a History of Applied Kinesiology," *Journal of Manipulative Physiological Therapeutics*, vol. 20, no. 5 (1997), pp. 331-337.
4. John Ankerberg and John Weldon, *Can You Trust Your Doctor?* (Brentwood, TN: Wolgemuth and Hyatt, 1991), pp. 157, 167.
5. George J. Goodheart, letter to author, February 17, 1999.
6. Gin and Green, "George Goodheart, Jr., D.C., and a History of Applied Kinesiology," pp. 331-337.
7. Dr. Goodheart, "Applied Kinesiology Is:," *International College of Applied Kinesiology Home Page*, 2002. http://www.icak.com/akis/AKis.html?44,10 (accessed May 10, 2002).
8. B. Klinkoski and C. Leboeuf, "A Review of the Research Papers Published by the International College of Applied Kinesiology from 1981 to 1987," *Journal of Manipulative Physiological Therapeutics*, vol. 13, no. 4 (1990), pp. 190-194.
9. Tom and Carole Valentine, *Applied Kinesiology: Muscle Response in Diagnosis, Therapy and Preventive Medicine* (Rochester, VT: Healing Arts Press, 1987), pp. 29, 117.
10. Gin and Green, "George Goodheart, Jr., D.C., and a History of Applied Kinesiology," pp. 331-337.
11. M. Haas et al., "Muscle Testing Response to Provocative Vertebral Challenge and Spinal Manipulation: A Randomized Controlled Trial of Construct Validity," *Journal of Manipulative Physiological Therapeutics*, vol. 17, no. 3 (1994), pp. 141-148.
12. M. Haas et al., "Responsiveness of Leg Alignment Changes Associated with Articular Pressure Testing to Spinal Manipulation: The Use of a Randomized Clinical Trial Design to Evaluate a Diagnostic Test with a Dichotomous Outcome," *Journal of Manipulative Physiological Therapeutics*, vol. 16, no. 5 (1993), pp. 306-311.
    M. Haas et al., "Reactivity of Leg Alignment to Articular Pressure Testing: Evaluation of a Diagnostic Test Using a Randomized Crossover Clinical Trial Approach," *Journal of Manipulative Physiological Therapeutics*, vol. 16, no. 4 (1993), pp. 220-227.

13. A. Lawson and L. Calderon, "Interexaminer Agreement for Applied Kinesiology Manual Muscle Testing," *Perceptual and Motor Skills,* vol. 84, no. 2 (1997), pp. 539-546.

14. J. J. Kenney, R. Clemens and K. D. Forsythe, "Applied Kinesiology Unreliable for Assessing Nutrient Status," *Journal of the American Dietetic Association,* vol. 88, no. 6 (1988), pp. 698-704.

15. George J. Goodheart, letter to author, February 17, 1999.

16. Dr. Goodheart, "Applied Kinesiology Is Not!!" *International College of Applied Kinesiology Home Page,* 2002. http://www.icak.com/akis/AKis.html?44,10 (accessed May 10, 2002).

17. Valentine, *Applied Kinesiology: Muscle Response in Diagnosis, Therapy and Preventive Medicine,* n.p.

18. Ankerberg and Weldon, *Can You Trust Your Doctor?* p. 167.

19. MTIA, *Protect: The Basic Care Bulletin,* The Philosophies Behind Modern Medical Practices, 2nd ed., 2 vols. (Oak Brook, IL: IBLP, 1996), pp. 14-15.

Chapter Seventeen

1. A. Tavani et al., "Margarine Intake and Risk of Nonfatal Acute Myocardial Infarction in Italian Women," *European Journal of Clinical Nutrition,* vol. 51, no. 1 (1997), pp. 30-32.

2. Rebecca Troisi, Walter C. Willett and Scott T. Weiss, "Trans-Fatty Acid Intake in Relation to Serum Lipid Concentrations in Adult Men," *American Journal of Clinical Nutrition,* vol. 56 (1992), pp. 1019-1024.

3. H. H. Vorster et al., "Dietary Cholesterol—the Role of Eggs in the Prudent Diet," *South Africa Medical Journal,* vol. 85, no. 4 (1995), pp. 253-256.

4. Robert C. Atkins, *Dr. Atkins' Diet Revolution* (New York: Bantam Books, 1972), p. 5.

5. Kevin V. Ergil, "China's Traditional Medicine," in *Fundamentals of Complementary and Alternative Medicine,* ed. Marc S. Micozzi (New York: Churchill Livingstone, 1995), pp. 185-223.

6. Elliot D. Abravanel and Elizabeth King Morrison, *Dr. Abravanel's Body Type Diet and Lifetime Nutrition Plan* (New York: Bantam Books, 1999), n.p.

7. Ben M. Edidin, *Jewish Customs and Ceremonies* (New York: Hebrew Publishing Company, 1941), pp. 33-42.

8. Walter Martin, *The Kingdom of the Cults* (Minneapolis, MN: Bethany House Publishers, 1965), pp. 360-423.

9. Rex Russell, *What the Bible Says About Healthy Living* (Ventura, CA: Regal Books, 1996), n.p.

10. Michael D. Jacobson, *The Word on Health: A Biblical and Medical Overview of How to Care for Your Body and Mind* (Chicago, IL: Moody Press, 2000), n.p.

11. Joseph E. Pizzorno, Jr., "Naturopathic Medicine," in *Fundamentals of Complementary and Alternative Medicine,* ed. Marc S. Micozzi (New York: Churchill Livingstone, 1995), pp. 163-181.

12. Elaine Gottschall, *Breaking the Vicious Cycle: Intestinal Health Through Diet* (Baltimore, Ontario: The Kirkton Press, 1994), n.p.

13. Margo Denke, "Dietary Fatty Acids and Atherosclerosis," *Lipids and Atherogenesis,* vol. 1, no. 1 (1991), pp. 4-7.

14. A. Keys, "Coronary Heart Disease in Seven Countries," *Circulation,* vol. 41, no. 1 (1970), pp. 1-211.
15. Anita B. Lasswell et al., *Nutrition and Cancer* (Hillsborough, NC: Medeor Interactive, 1998).
16. N. J. Gonzalez and L. L. Isaacs, "Evaluation of Pancreatic Proteolytic Enzyme Treatment of Adenocarcinoma of the Pancreas, with Nutrition and Detoxification Support," *Nutrition and Cancer,* vol. 33, no. 2 (1999), pp. 117-124.

   G. L. Hildenbrand et al., "Five-Year Survival Rates of Melanoma Patients Treated by Diet Therapy After the Manner of Gerson: A Retrospective Review," *Alternative Therapies in Health and Medicine,* vol. 1, no. 4 (1995), pp. 29-37.
17. Jacobson, *The Word on Health: A Biblical and Medical Overview of How to Care for Your Body and Mind,* pp. 70-76.
18. Russell, *What the Bible Says About Healthy Living,* n.p.
19. Dónal O'Mathúna and Walt Larimore, *Alternative Medicine: The Christian Handbook* (Grand Rapids, MI: Zondervan Publishing House, 2001), pp. 181-192.
20. Diane Hampton, *The Diet Alternative* (New Kensington, PA: Whitaker House, 1984), n.p.

Chapter Eighteen

1. Spiros Zodhiates, *Hebrew Greek Key Study Bible (King James Version),* ed. Spiros Zodhiates, 2nd ed. (Chattanooga, TN: AMG Publishers, 1991), p. 1533.
2. *Wycliffe Bible Commentary* (Willow Grove, PA: Woodlawn Electronic Publishing, 1988).
3. Brian Inglis and Ruth West, *The Alternative Health Guide* (New York: Alfred A. Knopf, 1983), p. 94.
4. Edward W. Cetaruk and Cynthia K. Aaron, "Hazards of Nonprescription Medications," *Emergency Medicine Clinics of North America,* vol. 12, no. 2 (1994), pp. 483-510.
5. Rudolf Fritz Weiss, *Herbal Medicine* (Gothenburg, Sweden: AB Arcanum, 1988), p. 8.
6. J. P. Davignon, L. A. Trissel and L. M. Kleinman, "Pharmaceutical Assessment of Amygdalin (Laetrile) Products," *Cancer Treatment Reports,* vol. 62, no. 1 (1978), pp. 99-104.
7. Weiss, *Herbal Medicine,* p. 7.
8. Brian Inglis, *A History of Medicine* (Cleveland, OH: The World Publishing Company, 1965), pp. 114-115.
9. *World Book Encyclopedia,* s.v. "vitamin."
10. Robert B. Baron, "Nutrition," in *Current Medical Diagnosis and Treatment,* ed. S. A. Schroeder et. al (Norwalk, CT: Appleton and Lange, 1990), pp. 859-890.
11. Anita B. Lasswell et al., *Nutrition and Cancer* (Hillsborough, NC: Medeor Interactive, 1998).
12. For more information, see excellent resources by Richard F. and Phyllis A. Balch, *Prescription for Nutritional Healing* (Garden City Park, NY: Avery Publishing Group, 1990) and Dónal O'Mathúna and Walt Larimore, *Alternative Medicine: The Christian Handbook* (Grand Rapids, MI: Zondervan Publishing House, 2001), which contain a summary of scientific literature on numerous natural remedies.

Chapter Nineteen

1. Dónal O'Mathúna and Walt Larimore, *Alternative Medicine: The Christian Handbook* (Grand Rapids, MI: Zondervan Publishing House, 2001), pp. 161-163.

2. Stephen A. Levine and Parris M. Kidd, *Antioxidant Adaptation* (Hayward, CA: Biocurrents Division, Allergy Research Group, 1986), pp. 16, 33.

3. E. F. Duhr et al., "HgEDTA Complex Inhibits GTP Interactions with the E-Site of Brain Beta-Tubulin," *Toxicology and Applied Pharmacology,* vol. 122, no. 2 (1993), pp. 273-280.

4. O. Torres-Alanis et al., "Urinary Excretion of Trace Elements in Humans after Sodium 2,3-Dimercaptopropane-1-Sulfonate Challenge Test," *Journal of Toxicology-Clinical Toxicology,* vol. 38, no. 7 (2000), pp. 697-700.

5. Elmer Cranton, *Bypassing Bypass* (Trout Dale, VA: Medex Publishers, 1993), pp. 75-81.

6. Harold Brecher and Arline Brecher, *Forty Something Forever: A Consumer's Guide to Chelation Therapy and Other Heart-Savers* (Herndon, VA: HealthSavers Press, 1992), pp. 241-248.

7. Benjamin N. Smith and Norman D. Grace, "Hemochromatosis," in *Conn's Current Therapy,* ed. Robert E. Rakel (Philadelphia, PA: W. B. Saunders Company, 1995), pp. 345-348.

8. E. Olszewer and J. P. Carter, "EDTA Chelation Therapy in Chronic Degenerative Disease," *Medical Hypotheses,* vol. 27, no. 1 (1988), pp. 41-49.

9. E. Ernst, "Chelation Therapy for Peripheral Arterial Occlusive Disease," *Circulation,* vol. 96, no. 3 (1997), p. 1031.

10. D. J. Green et al., "Effects of Chelation with EDTA and Vitamin B Therapy on Nitric Oxide-Related Endothelial Vasodilator Function," *Clinical and Experimental Pharmacology and Physiology,* vol. 26, no. 11 (1999), pp. 853-856.

11. Hal A. Huggins, *It's All in Your Head* (Garden City Park, NY: Avery Publishing Group, 1993), p. 23.

12. J. E. Dodes, "The Amalgam Controversy: An Evidence-Based Analysis," *Journal of the American Dental Association,* vol. 132, no. 3 (2001), pp. 348-356.

13. "Principles of Ethics and Code of Professional Conduct," *American Dental Association Home Page,* 2002. http://www.ada.org/prof/prac/law/code/opin05.html#5.A.1. (accessed May 2002).

14. IAOMT, "Achievements," *International Academy of Oral Medicine and Toxicology Home Page,* 2002. http://www.iaomt.org/where.htm (accessed May 9, 2002).

15. Huggins, *It's All in Your Head,* p. 23.

16. J. W. Reinhardt, "Side-Effects: Mercury Contribution to Body Burden from Dental Amalgam," *Advanced Dental Research,* vol. 6 (1992), pp. 110-113.

    L. Soleo et al., "The Influence of Amalgam Fillings on Urinary Mercury Excretion in Subjects from Apulia (Southern Italy)," *Giornale Italiano Medicina del Lavoro del Ergonomia,* vol. 20, no. 2 (1998), pp. 75-81.

17. F. L. Lorscheider, M. J. Vimy and A. O. Summers, "Mercury Exposure from 'Silver' Tooth Fillings: Emerging Evidence Questions a Traditional Dental Paradigm," *Faseb Journal,* vol. 9, no. 7 (1995), pp. 504-508.

    M. F. Ziff, "Documented Clinical Side-Effects to Dental Amalgam," *Advanced Dental Research,* vol. 6 (1992), pp. 131-134. This article explains that mercury exposure from dental amalgam occurs at a rate of anywhere from one- to sixfold greater than exposure from dietary sources.

18. E. Henriksson, U. Mattsson and J. Hakansson, "Healing of Lichenoid Reactions Following Removal of Amalgam: A Clinical Follow-Up," *Journal of Clinical Periodontology*, vol. 22, no. 4 (1995), pp. 287-294.

   Y. Finkelstein et al., "The Enigma of Parkinsonism in Chronic Borderline Mercury Intoxication, Resolved by Challenge with Penicillamine," *Neurotoxicology*, vol. 17, no. 1 (1996), pp. 291-295.

   D. McComb, "Occupational Exposure to Mercury in Dentistry and Dentist Mortality," *Journal of the Canadian Dental Association*, vol. 63, no. 5 (1997), pp. 372-376.

   J. S. Vamnes et al., "Diagnostic Value of a Chelating Agent in Patients with Symptoms Allegedly Caused by Amalgam Fillings," *Journal of Dental Research*, vol. 79, no. 3 (2000), pp. 868-874.

   A. K. Furhoff et al., "A Multidisciplinary Clinical Study of Patients Suffering from Illness Associated with Release of Mercury from Dental Restorations. Medical and Odontological Aspects," *Scandinavian Journal of Primary Health Care*, vol. 16, no. 4 (1998), pp. 247-252.

   S. Stenman and L. Grans, "Symptoms and Differential Diagnosis of Patients Fearing Mercury Toxicity from Amalgam Fillings," *Scandinavian Journal of Work Environment and Health*, vol. 23, no. 3 (1997), pp. 59-63.

   J. Bailer et al., "Adverse Health Effects Related to Mercury Exposure from Dental Amalgam Fillings: Toxicological or Psychological Causes?" *Psychological Medicine*, vol. 31, no. 2 (2001), pp. 255-263.

19. G. Sandborgh-Englund et al., "Mercury in Biological Fluids After Amalgam Removal," *Journal of Dental Research*, vol. 77, no. 4 (1998), pp. 615-624.

   C. C. Leong, N. I. Syed and F. L. Lorscheider, "Retrograde Degeneration of Neurite Membrane Structural Integrity of Nerve Growth Cones Following in Vitro Exposure to Mercury," *Neuroreport*, vol. 12, no. 4 (2001), pp. 733-737.

   C. Hock et al., "Increased Blood Mercury Levels in Patients with Alzheimer's Disease," *Journal of Neural Transmission*, vol. 105, no. 1 (1998), pp. 59-68.

   C. H. Ngim and G. Devathasan, "Epidemiologic Study on the Association Between Body Burden Mercury Level and Idiopathic Parkinson's Disease," *Neuroepidemiology*, vol. 8, no. 3 (1989), pp. 128-141.

   D. Bangsi et al., "Dental Amalgam and Multiple Sclerosis: A Case-Control Study in Montreal, Canada," *International Journal of Epidemiology*, vol. 27, no. 4 (1998), pp. 667-671.

   R. L. Siblerud and E. Kienholz, "Evidence That Mercury from Silver Dental Fillings May Be an Etiological Factor in Multiple Sclerosis," *Science of the Total Environment*, vol. 142, no. 3 (1994), pp. 191-205.

20. Ted J. Kaptchuk, "Historical Context of the Concept of Vitalism in Complementary and Alternative Medicine," in *Fundamentals of Complementary and Alternative Medicine*, ed. Marc S. Micozzi (New York: Churchill Livingstone, 1995), pp. 35-48.

21. O'Mathúna and Larimore, *Alternative Medicine: The Christian Handbook*, pp. 240-244.

22. Ibid.

23. Paul C. Reisser, Dale Mabe and Robert Velarde, *Examining Alternative Medicine: An Inside Look at the Benefits and Risks* (Downers Grove, IL: InterVarsity Press, 2001), p. 222.

24. Victoria E. Slater, "Healing Touch," in *Fundamentals of Complementary and Alternative Medicine*, ed. Marc S. Micozzi (New York: Churchill Livingstone, 1995), pp. 121-136.

25. Ibid., p. 122.

26. Ibid., pp. 121-122.
27. Reisser, Mabe and Velarde, *Examining Alternative Medicine: An Inside Look at the Benefits and Risks,* pp. 221-233.
28. O'Mathúna and Larimore, *Alternative Medicine: The Christian Handbook,* pp. 266-268.
29. D. P. Wirth and J. R. Cram, "Multisite Surface Electromyography and Complementary Healing Intervention: A Comparative Analysis," *Journal of Alternative and Complementary Medicine,* vol. 3, no. 4 (1997), pp. 355-364.
30. O'Mathúna and Larimore, *Alternative Medicine: The Christian Handbook,* pp. 244-246.
31. L. Rosa et al., "A Close Look at Therapeutic Touch," *Journal of the American Medical Association,* vol. 279, no. 13 (1998), pp. 1005-1010.

Chapter Twenty

1. Rollin McCraty, "Stress and Emotional Health" (paper presented at the Steroid Hormones Clinical Correlates: Therapeutic and Nutritional Considerations, Chicago, IL, February 25, 1996).
2. Hans Selye, *The Stress of Life* (New York: McGraw-Hill, 1956), n.p.
3. Michael D. Jacobson, *The Word on Health: A Biblical and Medical Overview of How to Care for Your Body and Mind* (Chicago, IL: Moody Press, 2000), n.p.
4. Archibald D. Hart, *Adrenalin and Stress* (Waco, TX: Word Books, 1986), p. 67.
5. McCraty, "Stress and Emotional Health."
6. Dónal O'Mathúna and Walt Larimore, *Alternative Medicine: The Christian Handbook* (Grand Rapids, MI: Zondervan, 2001), pp. 158-160, 246-249, 283-285.
7. *Dorland's Illustrated Medical Dictionary,* 26th ed., s.v. "hypnosis."
8. Ted J. Kaptchuk, "Historical Context of the Concept of Vitalism in Complementary and Alternative Medicine," in *Fundamentals of Complementary and Alternative Medicine,* ed. Marc S. Micozzi (New York: Churchill Livingstone, 1995), pp. 35-48.
9. O'Mathúna and Larimore, *Alternative Medicine: The Christian Handbook,* pp. 158-161.
10. L. Bernardi et al., "Effect of Rosary Prayer and Yoga Mantras on Autonomic Cardiovascular Rhythms: Comparative Study," *British Medical Journal,* vol. 323, no. 7327 (2001), pp. 1446-1449.
11. The Steps to Freedom in Christ is a tool developed by Freedom in Christ Ministries to help people resolve their personal and spiritual conflicts through repentance and faith in God. This tool (available in many forms) can be purchased through any Christian bookstore or from the Freedom in Christ Ministries website at http://www.ficm.org.

Chapter Twenty-One

1. Neil T. Anderson, *Released from Bondage* (Nashville, TN: Thomas Nelson, Inc., 2002), n.p.

GLOSSARY

acupressure—The Chinese practice of applying pressure to specific points on the body surface to relieve pain, induce anesthesia or treat various disorders by effecting changes in energy flow (qi).

acupuncture—The Chinese practice of inserting needles at specific points on the body surface to relieve pain, induce anesthesia or treat various disorders by effecting changes in energy flow (qi).

allopathy—A therapeutic approach rooted in Greek medicine that treats diseases by producing an antagonistic condition to what is to be cured and/or alleviated in the body.

animal magnetism—A hypothetical magnetic force believed by Austrian physician Frank Anton Mesmer to permeate all living beings and which can supposedly be manipulated with the practitioner serving as a medium.

applied kinesiology—The diagnostic and treatment system invented by George Goodheart, D.C., that associates muscles with specific organs and equates weakness with dysfunction or disease.

auriculotherapy—The Chinese practice of inserting needles into the external ear in order to affect the flow of energy (qi) and thereby treat disorders elsewhere in the body.

Ayurveda—An ancient Indian system of medicine that emphasizes maintaining balance and harmony with the universe on both a material (physical) and immaterial (spiritual) level through optimum lifestyle and meditation.

biofeedback—The use of instruments to provide feedback on the body's autonomic activities such as breathing rates, blood pressure, skin temperature, muscle tension, etc.

chelation—The binding of a complex substance with metals into a ring-like formation. It is used extensively in alternative medicine to treat a host of different diseases (such as coronary artery disease, cancer and multiple sclerosis) that are thought by some alternative practitioners to be due in part to a build up of toxic heavy metals.

chiropractic—A therapeutic approach based upon the premise that disease is caused by misalignment of spinal segments, which are treated through manipulation.

cognitive therapy—A philosophy based on the understanding that people are doing what they are doing and feeling the way they feel because of what they have chosen to believe or think.

craniosacral therapy—A therapeutic approach developed by William Sutherland, D.O., that emphasizes the functional and motion relationships between the bones of the cranium (skull) and sacrum (base of the spine).

dowsing—The ancient practice of "divining" information from the immaterial realm by the use of an object such as a pendulum.

Eastern mysticism—A general term referring to ancient concepts (and their related practices) of universal cosmic energy originating from Eastern cultures (especially China and India).

electro acupuncture—A Western modification of traditional Chinese medicine in which an instrument is used to assess and/or electrically stimulate acupuncture points in order to reflexively affect other areas or organs.

emetics—Drugs that induce vomiting.

fight or flight response—The constellation of physiological effects (such as increased blood flow to muscles and the rise in rates of heartbeat, breathing and blood pressure) stimulated by adrenaline, which is released when an animal or human being perceives a threat.

five phases—An ancient Chinese concept that all matter exists in one of five phases (earth, metal, water, wood and fire) and that energy moves between these phases. In medicine, each phase is correlated with hollow and solid (yin and yang) organs.

guided imagery—The use of the imagination to visualize a specific purpose.

healing touch—A method of healing using the hands, developed by Janet Mentgen, a Colorado nurse. It is based upon the ancient belief in a universal healing energy.

holism—A philosophical approach introduced in the early 1900s by Jan Smuts of South Africa, which proposes that individuals and systems are more than the sum of their parts and that they can only be understood in the context of their whole immaterial and material being and their relations with one another. Currently, the term is used most often in alternative medicine to describe New Age mind-body relationships and/or to emphasize the needs of the total person—mental, emotional, physical, environmental. See also "wholism."

homeopathy—A therapeutic system that treats disease with very dilute substances, which reportedly cause similar symptoms as the disease when given in larger doses to healthy individuals.

humanistic medicine—A mechanistic philosophy of medicine that does not acknowledge existence of the supernatural realm.

humoralism—An ancient therapeutic system of Greek medicine that proposes that all disease results from an imbalance of the body's basic humors (fluids).

humors (fluids)—A Greek variation of an ancient Ayurvedic concept in which human beings are composed of four basic humors, or fluids (blood, phlegm, yellow bile and black bile).

hydrotherapy—The therapeutic use of water to treat ailments and disease.

hypnotism—The practice of inducing a passive state of mind in order to make an individual more amenable to the suggestions or commands of another.

iridology—A diagnostic system that uses the iris of the eye to evaluate the health of the entire individual.

magnetism (magnets)—The use of magnets to treat pain, ailments or disease through effecting changes in an individual's electromagnetic fields (see "animal magnetism").

manipulative therapy—A method of therapy in which the operator uses his or her hands to restore the musculoskeletal system (especially the spine) to normal position and motion.

mechanistic science—The segment of ideas and individuals in the scientific community that either ignore or deny the existence of the supernatural. Reality is believed to only exist in the physical realm.

mental telepathy—The transmission of thought between two individuals.

mesmerism (higher and lower)—The concept that the immaterial energy that gives life and health (see "vitalism") has either a spiritual character (higher mesmerism) or a more physical character (lower mesmerism).

mind-body medicine—A philosophy of medicine based on the belief that cognitive thought influences the body and physical health in general.

motion theory—The dislocation of a body part involving more than one segment and which causes the motion between the different segments to become dysfunctional.

moxibustion—The ancient Chinese practice of burning the dried and powdered leaves of *Artemesia vulgaris* on or near the skin to effect the movement of qi.

naturopathy—A therapeutic system that presupposes the causation of disease to be an accumulation of toxins and which uses natural methods (such as air, light, water, heat and diet) as treatment.

New Age—A social movement from the late twentieth century that incorporates beliefs from Eastern and American Indian traditions (such as holism, environmentalism, spiritualism and metaphysics).

nutriceutical—A vitamin, mineral or other naturally occurring substance that has been formulated to treat specific ailments or conditions.

osteopathy—A therapeutic system based on the theory that the body makes its own remedies against disease and other ailments when it is in normal structural relationship and has a healthy environment and proper nutrition.

passive therapy—Therapy that is applied to the patient without the patient's active involvement. For example, in physical therapy, passive modalities include deep heat, electrical stimulation and ultrasound versus active modalities that involve the patient exercising his or her own muscles.

pharmaceutical—A manufactured drug used for medicinal purposes.

polarity—The property of having poles or opposites.

polarity therapy—An adaptation of Eastern medicine by Austrian Randolph Stone who asserted that the body has five centers of energy, each corresponding with one of five phases (ether, air, fire, water and earth). Each pole, or center, controls various bodily functions. Good health is maintained by keeping the forces in balance. Disease, due to imbalance, is treated with manipulation, postural exercises and diet.

prana—The Ayurvedic or Hindu term for universal energy, akin to Chinese qi.

prolotherapy—A method of treatment for damaged connective tissue (ligaments, joint capsules, tendons) in which injection of a substance into the area of injury provokes an inflammatory response and thereby stimulates the body to repair the injury.

psychosomatic illness—An illness in the body (soma) that is considered to have its root cause in dysfunctional thinking and emotions (i.e., the psyche). Often used to refer to stress-related psychological illnesses such as anxiety, depression, anger and addictions.

purgatives—Drugs that induce diarrhea.

purification therapy—A therapeutic system which uses various modalities to purge the body of toxins.

qi (chee)—An energy, or life force, according to Taoist philosophy, that permeates the universe and all living beings, traveling throughout the body via channels (meridians).

qigong (chee goong)—The practice of applying an inner force through mental and breathing exercises in order to balance the qi (energy, or life force) of one's own body or that of another (emitted qi).

radiesthesia—The application of dowsing to medicine (see "dowsing"), to divine the diagnosis, treatment or both.

radionics—The use of instrumentation to practice radiesthesia.

reflexology—A therapeutic system that utilizes the soles of the feet for the diagnosis and treatment of disease of the entire body through stimulating energy meridians to related organs.

reflexotherapy—The practice of treating an area of the body by stimulating points or areas that are related to the affected area by neurological reflexes.

reiki—A hand-mediated energy healing technique from Japan.

rhabdomancy—The practice of divination by using rods and/or wands.

shiatsu massage—A Japanese version of Chinese acupressure, now a more developed form of massage therapy.

Tao—The cosmic force behind nature's order. It has two faces: yin and yang.

Taoism—An ancient Eastern religion/philosophy that asserts that the first cause of the universe is immaterial energy that permeates the universe and every living being. Optimum health is only achieved when one is in harmony with the universe and when an unhindered flow of energy travels from the universe to the individual and back to the cosmos again.

therapeutic touch— A method of healing using the hands, developed by Delores Krieger and Dora Kunz and based upon the ancient belief in a universal healing energy.

Touch For Health—A British adaptation of applied kinesiology.

touch therapies—The practice of using touch to treat illnesses through the manipulation of energy fields.

traditional Chinese medicine—A heterogeneous system of medicine that has materialized over at least two millennia and is rooted in ancient Taoist concepts. It emphasizes the importance of living a quiet, balanced life in harmony with the universe and with an unhindered flow of cosmic energy that permeates the universe and all living beings.

transcendental meditation—An ancient Vedic technique for reconnecting to or increasing one's level of awareness of universal energy, or "transcendental consciousness," by emptying the mind of all distracting thoughts (i.e., transcending conscious thought to a more simple state of awareness).

visualization—The practice of picturing in one's mind a peaceful scene or environment in order to become relaxed.

vitalism—The concept of an immaterial energy force that gives life and health to the physical (see "mesmerism").

wholism—A term used interchangeably with "holism" but sometimes used in conjunction with it for the purpose of distinguishing itself from the latter's use in New Age concepts in order to acknowledge the biblical nature of man—spirit, soul and body. It recognizes the significance of man's spirit and soul (i.e., the inner man) to reach optimum physical health (the outer man) and vice versa. See also "holism."

yin and yang—A fundamental concept in ancient Chinese philosophy referring to aspects of the universe that oppose and yet complement one another. Described as opposite sides of the same hill, yin represents the shaded, cooler, feminine, northern side with plants and animals that favor it while yang represents the warmer, masculine side, with the growth and life that favor a southern exposure.

yoga ("the path of yoga")—Hindu exercises of breath control and postures conducted for the purpose of gaining release from the bondage of karma (the teaching that one's station in life is dependent upon how one lived in their prior life) and rebirth.

SCRIPTURE INDEX

INDEX

ADDITIONAL RESOURCES

The Word On Health

*A Biblical and Medical Overview of
How to Care For Your Body and Mind*

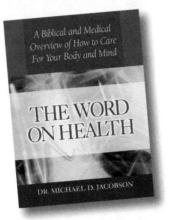

Whether Christian or secular, most books written on personal health tend to attribute today's illnesses to poor dietary habits. But Jesus never put anyone on a diet and very few if any of the Bible's promises of health and long life have anything to do with food. So, what does the Bible really have to say about how to attain optimum health?

In the first section, a foundation is laid that explains 7 biblical causes of illness, today's false dietary doctrines and how they are dividing families and churches, and a proper understanding of Christian liberty. The next section guides the reader through what the Bible *does* say about diet, and builds a Biblical Diet Pyramid strategy that has endured the test of time and much scientific validation. Finally, the book concludes with a powerful presentation of how spiritual problems become physical disease. The section includes an explanation of the myriad of effects that stress has on the body, the key role of the physical and spiritual heart, and steps to restoring spiritual, emotional and physical health.

This book will show you the timeless wisdom of God's Word and strengthen your faith. It is must reading for those who truly desire to understand the perspective the Bible brings to personal health. For many, it has become a standard by which other publications are evaluated. *The Word On Health* (©2000 Moody Press) is available in Christian bookstores and at www.providentmedical.com

Books and Tapes

Visit the books and tapes section at www.providentmedical.com or contact our ministry office for helpful resources available in print or on audio media. These include tape series on such topics as Women's Health, Spirit-Controlled Thoughts, Words & Emotions, The Word On Health Seminar, Conquering Addictions, Alternative Cancer Treatments and much more.

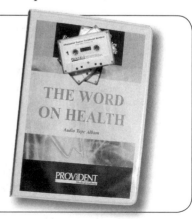

FROM DR. JACOBSON

Vital Signs

Vital Signs is a monthly newsletter designed by Provident Medical Institute to show the relevance of biblical faith to health and medicine. Each month features an in-depth biblical analysis of a current health concern in addition to brief reports on recent scientific breakthroughs and Dr. Jacobson's speaking schedule. Vital Signs is provided by e-mail and is available through our website or by contacting our office.

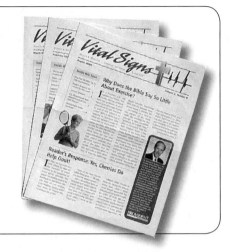

Speaking Opportunities

If you are interested in hosting Dr. Jacobson for a speaking event in your area, contact our office or visit our seminars website section.

Visit Our Ministry Web Site: www.providentmedical.com

- Learn more about Provident
- Subscribe to *Vital Signs* newsletter
- Free Med-Facts info-sheets on common medical problems

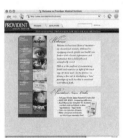

- Special sections for Pastors and Educators
- How to host a PMI Seminar
- Order page for a variety of PMI's books and tapes
- Dr. Jacobson's speaking schedule and seminar information

About Provident Medical Institute

Provident Medical Institute was established in 1995 for the purpose of glorifying Jesus Christ and strengthening the faith of His people through providing church and family leadership with health-related teaching that is Biblically and scientifically sound. PMI is a non-profit local church educational ministry.

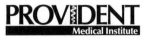 8501 Plainfield Road, Cincinnati, OH 45236
(513) 891-7925 www.providentmedical.com

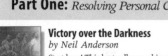
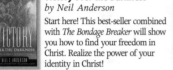

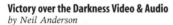

Freedom in Christ Resources

Part Three: *Discipleship Counseling*

Helping Others Find Freedom in Christ
by Neil Anderson

This book provides comprehensive, hands-on biblical discipleship counseling training for lay leaders, counselors and pastors, equipping them to help others.

Paperback $14.95 • 297 pp. B015
Training Manual and Study Guide $11.95

Helping Others Find Freedom in Christ Video Training Program

This Video Training Program is a complete training kit for churches and groups who want to establish a freedom ministry using *The Steps to Freedom in Christ*. Includes four 45-minute video lessons.

Video Training Program $39.95 • V015

Freedom from Addiction
by Neil Anderson and Mike and Julia Quarles

A book like no other on true recovery! This unique Christ-centered model has helped thousands break free from alcoholism, drug addiction and other addictive behaviors. The Quarles's amazing story will encourage every reader!

Paperback $16.95 • 356 pp. B019

Freedom from Addiction Video Study
by Neil Anderson and Mike and Julia Quarles

A dynamic resource for recovery group leading pastors and Christian counselors. A step-by-step study that changes lives. Includes video study, paperback and workbook.

Video Study $89.95 • V019

Discipleship Counseling
by Neil Anderson

This series presents advanced counseling insights and practical, biblical answers to help others find their freedom in Christ. It is the full content from Dr. Anderson's advanced seminar of the same name.

Videotape Set $99.95 • 8 lessons V033
Audiotape Set $44.95 • 8 lessons A033
Workbook $5 • Paper 24pp. W011

Setting Your Church Free
by Neil Anderson and Charles Mylander

This powerful book reveals how pastors and church leaders can lead their entire churches to freedom by discovering the key issues of both corporate bondage and corporate freedom. A must-read for every church leader.

Paperback $15.95 • 352 pp. B013

Part Four: *Church Leadership*

Setting Your Church Free Video Conference
by Neil Anderson and Charles Mylander

This leadership series presents the powerful principles taught in *Setting Your Church Free*. Ideal for church staffs and boards to study and discuss together. The series ends with the steps to setting your church free.

Videotape Set $69.95 • 8 lessons V006
Audiocassette Set $40 • 8 lessons A006
Additional workbooks $6 • paper 42 pp. W006
Corporate Steps $2 • G006

Topical Resources

God's Power at Work in You
by Neil Anderson and Robert Saucy

Anderson and Saucy deal with the dangerous common misconceptions that hinder spiritual growth, including: How can we overcome sin and resist temptation? What is God's role in helping us stay pure? What is our role? What is the key to consistent victory?

Paperback $10.95 B032

Released from Bondage
by Neil Anderson

This book shares true stories of freedom from obsessive thoughts, compulsive behaviors, guilt, satanic ritual abuse, childhood abuse and demonic strongholds, combined with helpful commentary from Dr. Anderson.

Paperback $12.95 • 258 pp. B006

Rivers of Revival
by Neil Anderson and Elmer Towns

Answers what many Christians are asking today: "What will it take to see revival?" Examines the fascinating subject of personal revival and past and current evangelistic streams that could help usher in global revival.

Hardcover $18.95 • 288 pp. B023

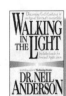

Walking in the Light
by Neil Anderson

Everyone wants to know God's will for his life. Dr. Anderson explains the fascinating spiritual dimensions of divine guidance and how to avoid spiritual counterfeits. Includes a personal application guide for each chapter.

Paperback $12.95 • 234 pp. B011

A Way of Escape
by Neil Anderson

Talking about sex is never easy. This vital book provides real answers for sexual struggles, unwanted thoughts, compulsive habits or a painful past. Don't learn to just cope; learn how to resolve your sexual issues in Christ.

Paperback $10.95 • 238 pp. B014

Freedom in Christ Resources

Topical Resources Continued

The Christ-Centered Marriage
by Neil Anderson and Charles Mylander

Husbands and wives, discover and enjoy your freedom in Christ together! Break free from old habit patterns and enjoy greater intimacy, joy and fulfillment.

Paperback $14.95 • 300 pp. B025

The Christ-Centered Marriage Video Seminar
by Neil Anderson and Charles Mylander

Everything you need in one package for setting marriages free in Christ. Thirteen short video discussion/starter segments enhance using the book and study guide. A great resource for pastors, Christian marriage counselors and Sunday School teachers.

Video Seminar $89.95 • V020

Marriage Steps • Paperback $6 • 3 Versions

Parenting Resources

Spiritual Protection for Your Children
by Neil Anderson and Peter and Sue VanderHook

The fascinating true story of an average middle-class American family's spiritual battle on the home front, and the lessons we can all learn about protecting our families from the enemy's attacks. Includes helpful prayers for children of various ages.

Paperback $12.95 • 300 pp. B021

The Seduction of Our Children
by Neil Anderson

This parenting book and series will change the way you view the spiritual development of your children. Helpful insights are offered on many parenting issues such as discipline, communication and spiritual oversight of children. A panel of experts share their advice.

Paperback $9.95 • 245 pp. B004
Videotape Set $59.95 • 6 lessons V004
Audiotape Set $35 • 6 lessons A004
Additional workbooks $4 • 49 pp. W004

Youth Resources

Stomping Out the Darkness
by Neil Anderson and Dave Park

This youth version of *Victory over the Darkness* shows youth how to break free and discover the joy of their identity in Christ. (Part 1 of 2.)

Paperback $9.95 • 210 pp. B101
Study Guide Paperback $8.95 • 137 pp. G101

The Bondage Breaker Youth Edition
by Neil Anderson and Dave Park

This youth best-seller shares the process of breaking bondages and the *Youth Steps to Freedom in Christ*. Read this with *Stomping Out the Darkness*. (Part 2 of 2.)

Paper $8.95 • 248 pp. B102
Study Guide Paper $6.95 • 128 pp. G102

Youth Resources Continued

Busting Free!
by Neil Anderson and Dave Park

This is a dynamic group study of *Stomping Out the Darkness* and *The Bondage Breaker Youth Edition*. It has complete teaching notes for a 13-week (or 26-week) Bible study, with reproducible handouts. Ideal for Sunday School classes, Bible studies and youth discipleship groups of all kinds.

Manual $16.95 • 163 pp. G103

Youth Topics

Leading Teens to Freedom in Christ
by Neil Anderson and Rich Miller

This youth version provides comprehensive, hands-on biblical discipleship counseling training for parents, youth workers and youth pastors, equipping them to help young people.

Paperback $12.95 • 300 pp. B112

Purity Under Pressure
by Neil Anderson and Dave Park

Real answers for real world pressures! Youth will find out the difference between being friends, dating and having a relationship. No hype, no big lectures; just straightforward talk about living free in Christ.

Paperback $8.95 • 200 pp. B104

Youth Devotionals

These four 40-day devotionals help young people understand God's love and their identity in Christ. Teens will learn to establish a positive spiritual habit of getting into God's Word on a daily basis.

Extreme Faith
Paperback $8.95
200 pp. B108

Awesome God
Paperback $8.95
200 pp. B108

Reality Check
Paperback $8.95
200 pp. B107

Ultimate Love
Paperback $8.95
209 pp. B109

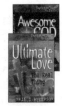

Real Life
Paperback $8.95
200 pp. B115

Sold Out for God
Paperback $8.95
200 pp. B116

Righteous Pursuit
Paperback $8.95
200 pp. B114

Biblically-Based Reading for Healthy Living

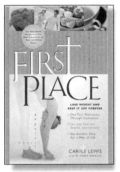

First Place
Lose Weight and
Keep It Off Forever
Carole Lewis with *Terry Whalin*
Paperback
ISBN 08307.28635

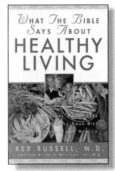

What the Bible Says About Healthy Living
Three Biblical Principles That
Will Change Your Diet and
Improve Your Health
Rex Russell, M.D.
Paperback
ISBN 08307.18583

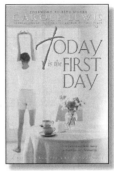

Today Is the First Day
Daily Encouragement on
the Journey to Weight
Loss and a Balanced Life
Carole Lewis,
General Editor
Hardcover
ISBN 08307.30656

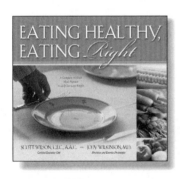

Eating Healthy, Eating Right
A Complete 16-Week Meal Planner
to Help You Lose Weight
Scott Wilson, C.I.C., A.A.C.
and *Jody Wilkinson* M.D.
Hardcover • ISBN 08307.30222

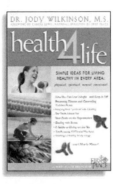

Health 4 Life
55 Simple Ideas for Living
Healthy in Every Area
Jody Wilkinson, M.D.
Paperback
ISBN 08307.30516

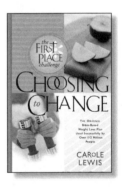

Choosing to Change
The First Place Challenge
Carole Lewis
Paperback
ISBN 08307.28627

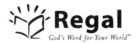